# LIVING WITH CHRONIC HEARTBURN

# LIVING WITH CHRONIC HEARTBURN

## *The Complete Health Guide to Acid Reflux & Gastroesophageal Reflux Disease (GERD)*

PAULO PACHECO, M.D.

and MARILYN OLSON

A HEALTHY LIVING BOOK

*New York • London*

# LIVING WITH CHRONIC HEARTBURN

Healthy Living Books
5-22 46th Avenue, Suite 200
Long Island City, NY 11101
1-800-528-2550
www.healthylivingbooks.com

DISCLAIMER
This book does not give legal or medical advice.
Always consult your doctor, lawyer, and other professionals.
The names of people who contributed anecdotal material have been changed.

Names of medications are typically followed by ™ or ® symbols, but these symbols are not stated in this book.

The ideas and suggestions contained in this book are not intended as a substitute for consulting with a physician. All matters regarding your health require medical supervision.

Library of Congress Cataloging-in-Publication Data

Pacheco, Paulo, M.D., 1967–
    Living with chronic heartburn : a guide for patients / Paulo Pacheco.
        p. cm.
    Includes bibliographical references.
    ISBN 1-57826-102-3 (alk. paper)
    1. Heartburn—Popular works. 2. Gastroesophageal reflux—Popular works. I. Title.

    RC 815.7. P23 2003
616. 3'2—dc21

                                                                          2003050865

All Hatherleigh Press titles are available for special promotions and premiums.
For more information, please call 1-800-528-2550 and ask for the manager of our Special Sales department.

Cover design by Tai Blanche
Printed in Canada on acid-free paper
10  9  8  7  6  5  4  3  2

*For Paul,*
*who always listens*
*and forever understands.*

# ACKNOWLEDGEMENTS

I'D LIKE TO THANK THE FOLLOWING PEOPLE WHO HELPED MAKE THIS book possible: Marilyn Olsen, who has been a tireless worker, advisor, and friend. Dr. Arnie Lambroza, for reviewing my manuscript and for his expert advice and friendship—thank you, Arnie. Dr. Dennis Fowler, for his time and advice regarding surgical options for reflux disease. New York Presbyterian Hospital–Weill Cornell nurses and technicians, for their support and help. My dear colleagues, both full-time and voluntary faculty and fellows, for their continued support. Dr. Carl McDougall, my new partner in private practice—thanks for your friendship, I look forward to working with you. Angela Acosta, my dear secretary; what can I say—you're wonderful.

To all my dear friends in New York and abroad (you know who you are)—thanks for listening to me at all hours of the day and for your advice, support, and friendship. Brad Meltzer and Cori Flam, my brilliant friends who are great writers and wonderful parents—thank you.

I'd also like to acknowledge the Brennan and Reed families for their love and friendship—Emily and James, I love you! My sister Angela—you've never let me down, you've always lifted me up; I love you. Her wonderful husband Arthur Cabral—you're one of the sweetest guys in the world. My two beautiful nieces Sara and Sofia—Uncle Paulo loves you! Fred and Deodete Pacheco, my wonderful parents, for all your love, time, energy, and support—I owe everything to you. And finally, Paul Brennan, whose faith and kindess never waivered. Thank you for your patience and support—without you, this book would not exist.

# CONTENTS

# FOREWORD

I F NOT QUITE UNIVERSAL, HEARTBURN IS A widespread human condition. To many people, an occasional episode of this symptom of acid reflux is a mere annoyance. However to others, it is a frequent occurrence that dramatically impairs quality of life. Heartburn is the most common manifestation of a condition that has come to be known as gastroesophageal reflux disease, or GERD, but many patients with GERD suffer from other symptoms that range from chest pain to difficulty swallowing to chronic cough and even asthma.

Several factors have led to intense focus on GERD among patients and physicians in recent years. The American diet is all too often rich in fatty or fried foods, which promote acid reflux directly. Even more importantly, being overweight predisposes one to reflux, and obesity is becoming increasingly prevalent in our society. Indeed, it is not uncommon for patients to consult a gastroenterologist for reflux—either new or worsened—that has accompanied weight gain.

The widespread availability of endoscopy has allowed physicians to assess the degree of acid-related injury to the esophageal lining. Our ability to treat acid reflux encompasses a wide assortment of medical treatments. They range from antacids to the older H2 receptor antagonists, which have been available over the counter for years, to the class of drugs called proton pump inhibitors, of which there are at least five presently on the market and which provide profound acid inhibition with remarkable safety. Finally, laparoscopy has offered a surgical alternative to open surgery as an operative approach to the problem, even as ingenious new techniques have been developed that can be applied through endoscopes without resorting to surgery at all.

A primary reason GERD has become one of the "hottest" topics in gastroenterology is the recognition of the role GERD plays in cancer of the esophagus. This dreaded disease is nearly always fatal when it presents with symptoms, such as food becoming stuck in the throat upon swallowing (there are benign cause of this symptom, as well). The link between GERD and cancer is a condition called Barrett's esophagus. This condition is characterized by a transformation of cells, called "metaplasia," in the lower esophagus from those that normally exist in that location to a very different type of cell—those that normally line the intestine. Barrett's esophagus develops in about 10 percent of people with chronic acid reflux, and may affect as little an inch or less of the lower esophagus (the area of maximal acid exposure in GERD) up to a large portion of the total length of the esophagus.

It has become increasingly common for gastroenterologists to perform endoscopy in people with longstanding reflux to identify those with Barrett's esophagus. People found to have this condition are then monitored periodically with endoscopy to identify any precancerous change in the esophageal lining cells, called dysplasia, before invasive cancer develops. Enormous attention is being devoted to the development of appropriate strategies for various degrees of dysplasia, especially high-grade or severe dysplasia, including the use of endoscopic techniques and medications as an alternative to surgery. Similarly, physicians would value any means of preventing the development of dysplasia in the first place with medications or endoscopy. There is as yet no universal consensus on how to achieve these goals, but this area remains one of intensive clinical research and lively controversy in gastroenterology.

Given the enormous importance of GERD in our society, a book on this topic intended for the general public is most timely. The present volume is a thorough, clearly written work that includes invaluable information on every aspect of this condition. People with GERD will take from this book a greatly enhanced understanding of their condition and what they need to do to cope successfully with it. There is a wealth of information about subjects ranging from medications used for GERD to the caloric content of many foods. Written in a lively, sympathetic, and engaging style, the book contains numerous "pearls" that are seldom found inside one cover. Topics like xercise, weight loss, and herbal or alternative therapies will be of interest to those with only occasional GERD or even no GERD at all. There are fascinating tidbits of history, ranging from the influence of the ancient physicians Hippocrates and Galen to the great English physician William Harvey and the date (1862) when the U.S. government began to regulate drugs. Physicians caring for patients with GERD should welcome books like this one, with its balanced approach and wealth of information, as an adjunct to their own efforts to control this important problem.

*Ira M. Jacobson, M.D.*
*Vincent Astor Professor of Clinical Medicine*
*Chief, Division of Gastroenterology and Hepatology*
*Weill Medical College of Cornell University*

# 1

# WHAT IS HEARTBURN?
## *An Introduction*

HEARTBURN IS THE MOST COMMON OF ALL human digestive complaints. What we eat, how we eat, and the condition of our digestive system are all factors that have contributed to the prevalence of heartburn throughout human history. And although we commonly call the condition "heartburn," that's really a misnomer, since it is a condition that affects the upper digestive system rather than the heart. A more appropriate term for the disease is GERD, the acronym for gastroesophageal reflux disease. Simply put, GERD occurs when something gastric (from the stomach) backs up (refluxes) into the esophagus. This happens to virtually everyone at some time or other and to some of us on a regular and frequent basis. In fact, it is estimated that 65 percent of the United States population has suffered from GERD at some time. Ten percent of us suffer from it on a weekly basis and 30 percent on a monthly basis. Twenty-four percent of those who have it have had symptoms for more than 10 years. These are only estimates because it is also generally believed that although GERD is a common problem in the

United States, the majority of people with the disease do not seek medical attention or report its symptoms to a doctor.

GERD typically is caused by the relaxation of the lower esophageal sphincter (LES), a muscle at the base of the esophagus where the esophagus connects with the stomach. (We'll discuss the causes of this relaxation in Chapter 2.) GERD can also be caused by a rupture of the diaphragm (the large muscle in the abdomen that normally surrounds the LES). Such a rupture is called a hiatal hernia, a condition that can occur as we age or during pregnancy.

Despite the frequency with which the disease occurs, many physicians and patients alike fail to recognize and diagnose GERD. One reason for this failure lies in the misconception that all GERD patients experience classic heartburn symptoms. Heartburn, though it is a major symptom of GERD, is only one of a long list of potential symptoms that patients may experience. Many patients have profound symptoms that are more severe than those of heartburn.

GERD is experienced by different people in different ways. For many it is an occasional problem that is simply endured or cleared up with over-the-counter antacids. For others, the disease occurs frequently, several times a week. For yet others, GERD, whether occasional or frequent is intensely painful. And, for the truly unfortunate, GERD is chronic. It occurs all the time; day after day, month after month, year after year. Yet, often, even people who experience GERD all the time fail to consult a physician and have these "benign" symptoms for many years even when the symptoms adversely affect eating, sexual activity, and interactions with others.

## *History of GERD*

GERD has probably plagued humanity since the first cavemen settled back to relax after an overly ambitious dinner of tasty, but greasy, mastodon. We know for sure that it was a problem for the early Romans. The historian Pliny the Elder, perhaps a sufferer himself, left a written record of his recommended remedy—coral powder. No doubt it did give him some relief because coral powder is mostly calcium carbonate, the main ingredient in the antacids used today.

Second century Greek physician Galen is credited with giving the disease its name kardialgia, "heart pain." Galen's prescription for relief was probably even more effective than Pliny's: Opium was a main ingredient among the 70 or more compounds in the concoction he brewed. Not content to stick with the tried and true, and perhaps discouraged by the fact that no matter what they did the symptoms kept recurring, over the centuries healers of varying degrees of education and competence tried herbs, spells, narcotics, and a perennial cure-all of historic medicine, leeches.

By the early 1800s, however, most physicians were suggesting a diet of bland food, milk, and antacids, still without coming up with a "cure" for the underlying problem.

Perhaps the most noted advocate of a diet regimen was early twentieth-century doctor Bertram Sippy. Determined to cure heartburn once and for all, Sippy confined his patients to bed for a month, giving them nothing but milk, antacids, eggs, and cereal. While no doubt many of his test subjects experienced welcome relief from heartburn, a good many of them found the program more effective as a weight-loss plan. A contemporary newspaper story reported that one of Sippy's patients escaped from the hospital. Wearing only her hospital gown, she walked across the street to a diner, consumed a full turkey dinner, and declaired that she would rather die from heartburn than starve to death.

## GERD Today

In most television commercials GERD is portrayed primarily as a disease of middle age. Actually, however, people of all ages experience it. Since its symptoms often resemble those of other diseases, it is often misdiagnosed. An especially nasty episode of GERD, for example, can feel like a heart attack.

Even though GERD as we now know it has existed for centuries, the greatest body of literature to emerge on this disease has materialized in the past 10 to 15 years. In fact, a great deal of interest in GERD has recently appeared in medical literature because of its documented relationship to Barrett's esophagus (a condition that can be a precursor to cancer) and other complications among chronic GERD sufferers who remain untreated.

In addition to feeling pretty scary, GERD can actually be pretty scary. Although the human stomach is fully equipped to handle stomach acid (more about that in the next chapter) the esophagus is not. When stomach acid, which is every bit as corrosive as the acid in the battery of a car, hits the tender lining of the esophagus, it is certain to cause trouble.

A frequent misconception about GERD is that patients with the condition have higher levels of acid production in the stomach (and therefore in the esophagus) than those who do not suffer from GERD. This has not been shown to be the case. In fact, quite the opposite may be true. Often GERD sufferers actually produce less stomach acid. The main problem is not the amount of acid, but the fact that the acid is entering an area (the esophagus) that is not designed to tolerate acid exposure. Therefore, any amount of acid can be corrosive and damaging.

For some people GERD is an unwelcome but temporary inconvenience; for millions of Americans, it is not just painful and debilitating, it is expensive as well. It is estimated that Americans spend $3 billion annually trying to control GERD and other digestive upsets.

Both acute (new) and chronic GERD can interrupt sleep, social interactions, work, sexual relations, and day-to-day activities. It is a common disorder that usually does not result in serious long-term consequences but can be overlooked by patients and physicians, particularly if patients fail to discuss it with their doctor.

If untreated, patients with chronic GERD can suffer serious long-term effects that can lead to shorter life (due primarily to cancer) or increased morbidity (esophageal scarring and narrowing). All patients who have frequent symptoms of GERD should therefore be evaluated by a gastroenterologist. Patients who wait too long to be treated may have esophageal injuries resulting in erosions (small injuries to the esophageal lining), ulcerations, bleeding, strictures (narrowing in the esophagus from chronic scarring), Barrett's esophagus (which we'll discuss later), and cancer. These complications can occur in patients with or without symptoms of reflux.

Certainly we know much more about how our bodies work than the ancient Greeks or even the physicians of the last century. We also have an arsenal of medications, surgeries, and lifestyle regimens that can in most cases lead to a cure or alleviation of most symptoms. We still can't treat patients, however, who don't tell us they have a problem.

If you have experienced any of the symptoms described in Chapter 3 or just want to make sure that acid reflux is not causing harm to your esophagus, see your doctor.

We're hopeful that reading this book will be the first step you take in helping yourself and your doctor come to terms with the problem of GERD in your life.

## Searching for a Cure

Today we are generally healthier than our ancestors thanks to antibiotics, early diagnosis, vaccines, and a host of sophisticated medical tests, but our bodies still function in much the same way they did in the Neanderthal era. Our dependence on junk food and fast food may be harder on our digestive systems than mastadon meat.

Is there a cure? We think we're getting closer. If you are reading this book, you probably have a personal interest in acid reflux and are looking for a solution to the problem. In the pages that follow you will learn more about the disease you share with one in three Americans. You will learn about the latest theories about the causes of this disease and what the medical community is doing to effect a cure. No leeches, we promise.

We're hopeful that as you learn more about GERD, you will find the combination of lifestyle changes, medication, and procedures that work best for you.

# 2

# UNDERSTANDING
# DIGESTION
## *An Overview*

To understand the causes of gerd, it's helpful to understand how the digestive process works.

The digestive system is one long tube that begins at the mouth and ends at the anus. Attached to this tube are digestive glands (the liver, gallbladder and pancreas) that secrete enzymes, which are proteins that break food down into nutrients that can be absorbed by the bloodstream.

Digestion begins in the mouth. As food is chewed, the salivary glands secrete saliva, which lubricates food so it can easily flow down the throat. Saliva also contains an enzyme, amylase, that begins to break down starch. The teeth crush the food into pieces of manageable size and the tongue forms the food into a ball (called a bolus) that can be easily swallowed.

Just prior to swallowing, the back of the tongue pushes the bolus into the esophagus while the soft palate closes off the passage to the nose and epiglottis (a flap on the top of the trachea) to keep food from entering your lungs. The esophagus serves as the transport system from the mouth to the rest of the digestive system for the solids and liquids essential to life, making it vital to the digestive process.

The upper esophageal sphincter (UES) is a muscle that relaxes following the upward movement of the hyoid bone (a horseshoe shaped bone at the base of the tongue and larynx). The movement of the hyoid bone acts as a stimulus that stretches the esophagus. If this stimulus is not well coordinated, pain and discomfort can occur.

Once the food is swallowed (i.e., has entered the esophagus), the UES closes to maintain atmospheric pressure in the esophagus and to keep the food from escaping back into the mouth. Then the food begins to move down the esophagus toward the stomach.

The esophagus is about 12 inches (30 centimeters) long and is composed of striated and smooth muscle tissue. Striated muscle is mainly attached to bones and allows for voluntary muscle control. Smooth muscle moves automatically under the control of the autonomic nervous system. In humans, the proportion of striated to smooth muscle changes, from 5 percent smooth muscle at the top of the esophagus to around 60 percent where the esophagus joins the stomach.

Both the striated and smooth muscle tissues contain nerves. These nerves stimulate the muscles in the esophagus to begin to move solids and liquids downward toward your stomach in a contracting and relaxing motion called peristalsis. Primary peristalsis is initiated by swallowing. Peristalsis in the rest of your esophagus is initiated by movement in any part of it. During peristalsis, the esophagus may lengthen or shorten by two to two and a half centimeters. Good digestion depends on even peristaltic motion.

In addition to pushing solids and liquids down toward the stomach, the esophagus also moves air. Swallowing too much air (or other substances such as cigarette smoke) can also cause problems in this part of the digestive system.

When food reaches the bottom of the esophagus, the lower esophageal sphincter (LES) opens, allowing the solids and liquids to enter the stomach. The LES then closes (or is supposed to close) to keep the solids and liquids in the stomach so the digestive process can continue.

**Figure 2A**

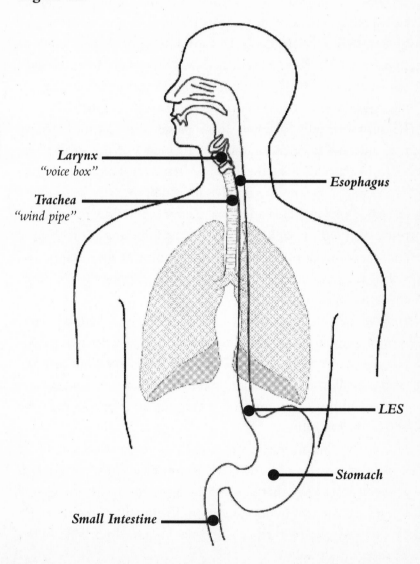

Larynx "voice box"

Trachea "wind pipe"

Esophagus

LES

Stomach

Small Intestine

Sensing that there is nothing more on the way, the LES and the UES remain closed to keep the esophagus empty. When one or both of the sphincters are not functioning properly, food or liquid remains in or re-enters the esophagus producing the symptoms of GERD.

The entrance of food into the stomach stimulates it to begin producing stomach acid. The muscles in the wall of the stomach also constrict and relax, compacting the food into even smaller pieces as the stomach acid begins to break it down chemically into nutrients that can be absorbed by the intestines. When the stomach is empty it no longer produces acid and contractions cease. (See figure 2A)

The now partially digested food passes through the pyloric sphincter into the duodenum, the first 10 inches of the small intestine. Here, bile produced by the liver is secreted through the gall bladder via the bile duct into the duodenum. Bile primarily helps digest fats. Digestive enzymes created by the pancreas also flow through the pancreatic duct out through an opening called the ampulla where the bile duct meets it. All of these enzymes combine as they empty into the wall of the small intestine. Pancreatic enzymes help break down carbohydrates, proteins and fats.

While all this is happening, the muscles of the small intestine contract, crushing the food into smaller and smaller particles that gradually become absorbed by various complex carrier methods into the wall of the small intestine and are transported into the bloodstream. It takes three to five hours for food to travel from your mouth to the end of the small intestine.

Once in the bloodstream, the nutrients go to the liver. Once there, some are stored and others are transformed into compounds that are transported to other parts of the body to supply energy and fuel for all cellular and bodily functions. Eventually these nutrients make their way to individual cells and the cells feed off these nutrients to sustain themselves.

Undigested food passes on to the large intestine (colon) where the water is squeezed out and absorbed and the semi-solid waste is expelled through the anus.

## What Can Go Wrong?

Since GERD-related illnesses occur in the upper gastrointestinal tract, we will now confine our discussion to the disorders that happen between the mouth and the entrance to the small intestine.

Both the esophagus and stomach contain strong muscles and nerves that stimulate them to constrict and relax, forcing food to travel from the mouth toward the stomach. That movement is called peristalsis. In most cases these muscles work so well that the digestive process can go on successfully even if people are upside down or floating weightless in outer space. The combination of the muscles and valves keep everything where it is supposed to be. As powerful as these muscles and valves are, however, they are designed to move things in one direction only. When what they are trying to move goes the other way, problems occur. Since digestion is a continuous process, even a minor mishap can throw the system off.

Fortunately for us, our brains have been programmed with a great many contingency plans. When anything does go wrong, our brain instantly moves on to "Plan B." If we touch something hot, we reflexively pull our hands away. If we see something frightening, a release of adrenaline allows us to run in the other direction. And, when anything moves in the wrong direction in our digestive system, our body immediately tries to correct the situation.

If a chunk of food inadvertently gets lodged in our throat, our body tries try to dislodge it with a cough. If we get the giggles while drinking milk, our body will send the milk out through our nose so we won't choke on it. If we eat or drink too much of the wrong food our medulla oblongata sends a message to our stomach that makes us vomit it up before it poisons us.

As unpleasant as all these "Plan B" reactions may be at the time, they exist for our own good. Most "Plan B" events are quickly over and forgotten with little harm done.

Unfortunately, other problems can occur. Some do no appreciable good and others last much longer than any of us would want. Some of these problems are congenital, that is, they have existed since birth. They include malformations of the esophagus or sphincters that open and close to allow food to pass through the esophagus into the stomach; nerve or muscle abnormalities that interfere with the ability of the esophagus or stomach to contract correctly; or growths that can cause blockages.

Some problems, such as scarring or tumors, develop over time. Others occur as a side effect of other diseases such as asthma or obesity. Still other problems result from diseases that occur primarily in the esophagus (e.g., achalasia) or diseases that are considered autoimmune (e.g., scleroderma). Patients often develop esophogeal problems later in life that can disturb their digestion such as scarring or tumor formation. Side effects of alcohol use, cigarette smoking, coffee, medication, and other dietary and lifestyle factors can all contribute to esophageal disorders.

Whatever the reason or cause may be, the result will likely be GERD. And that's what this book is all about.

# 3

# SYMPTOMS OF GERD
## *Recognizing the Warning Signs*

ECAUSE GERD IS A DISEASE OF THE UPPER intestinal tract, its symptoms occur primarily in the upper chest, throat, and mouth. Although symptoms such as bloating, diarrhea, and gas are also indications of intestinal disturbances, they are usually signs of upsets of the stomach or intestines.

The symptoms of GERD appear about equally among both men and women as well as in infants and children. The following are the symptoms that often lead to a diagnosis of GERD.

### Chest Pain

Chest discomfort can mimic heart disease and range from mild to severe in nature. Patients may experience their first attack of reflux in the middle of the night, with severe crushing chest pain that can cause intense anxiety and concern. Others may feel intermittent discomfort that is barely noticeable. Actually, these patients are often of most concern to doctors because they are less likely to seek medical attention while they keep taking over-the-counter preparations for extended periods of time. Since these medicines often help alleviate the symptoms, patients often decide not to consult their doctor.

## Heartburn and Its Triggers

One of the most common GERD symptoms is a burning sensation that seems to radiate out from the center of the chest, which is why the term heartburn was and is still used to identify GERD. Remember, however, GERD and heartburn are not synonymous. Only about two-thirds of all patients with GERD have heartburn. (In the remaining third, other symptoms predominate.)

Neither GERD nor heartburn is related to heart disease, but GERD can produce symptoms that are so painful they can provoke angina or other types of underlying heart disease. It is therefore important to pay close attention to symptoms and to seek medical attention if those GERD symptoms occur in an atypical fashion. GERD can be a serious mimicker of cardiac disease. In fact, more than 50 percent of patients with angina type chest pain are found to have GERD, once cardiac-related causes for their symptoms are ruled out. If there is any question about what your symptoms may mean, you should seek medical attention.

The burning sensation seen in reflux disease can be triggered by one or more of the following:

- *Consuming alcoholic beverages*
- *Consuming beverages or foods high in caffeine*
- *Consuming carbonated beverages*
- *Eating large meals*
- *Eating or drinking "on the run"*
- *Eating or drinking on an irregular schedule*
- *Eating unusual or spicy foods*
- *Lying down or going to bed soon after eating or drinking*

Other factors that may exacerbate symptoms include:

- *Excess intake of chocolate*
- *High fat foods*
- *Medications*

- *Peppermint/spearmint*
- *Tobacco*

GERD symptoms are often worsened by factors such as lying down and leaning over and bringing one's head below the waistline.

For most people, the burning sensation is uncomfortable but mild enough that symptoms disappear after a short time, either on their own or after taking an antacid. For other people, however, the burning sensation is very intense and it frequently occurs or lasts for a long time. It is important to know that even mild symptoms, over a long period of time, can result in consequences that can be serious to your digestive health and well-being. Early intervention and treatment can prevent long-term irreversible damage to your esophagus.

SOUR MOUTH Sour mouth is a nasty taste in the mouth resulting from the reflux of acids into the esophagus. The medical term for this is water brash. Water brash typically results from hyper-salivation (too much salivation) caused by chronic exposure of the esophagus to acid. The result can be a sudden, very acidic taste in your mouth, which is another common symptom of GERD. Sometimes the symptom lasts for just a few seconds following eructation (a burp) or a cough. Other times, this sour taste can last for hours at a time. This symptom is often worse in those who have multiple factors contributing to the reflux event, such as smoking or alcohol consumption.

STRESS Although stress has not been scientifically proven to be a direct cause of reflux disease, it has been shown that stress reduction can improve the outcome in patients with this disease.

## Pulmonary Symptoms

ASTHMA Asthma is a condition that can often be induced by acid reflux disease. The symptom may be a wheeze, which can be mild or moderate to severe and may also be associated with a chronic cough. In patients with GERD, asthma need not be treated with asthma preparations. Oftentimes treatment of GERD will be sufficient when combined with either lifestyle modifications or antacid preparations.

HICCUPS Although not a proven result of GERD in adults, up to 36 percent of infants can have daily hiccups that are thought to be related to reflux. There is some speculation that mechanoreceptor stimulation (receptors in the esophagus that are sensitive differences in pressure or touch) can cause hiccups, but no direct evidence exists that supports acid reflux as a causative factor for hiccups.

LARYNGEAL AND VOICE DISORDERS GERD has been shown to affect many functions of the laryngeal system. For example, chronic acid regurgitation can lead to laryngitis or hoarseness (reflux laryngitis) resulting in a raspy voice that will not subside.

Other symptoms include a sore throat, which is usually a result of reflux pharyngitis. This symptom is caused by acid that irritates the back of the throat (pharynx).

Excessive clearing of the throat is also sometimes seen in patients with GERD. This symptom is caused by direct acid reflux into the pharynx. A less common symptom is a persistent lump in the back of the throat (known as a globus sensation), a condition that may cause great concern in some patients. Sinusitis is another supra-esophageal (a symptom associated with, but not coming from within the esophagus) manifestation of GERD. The acid reflux can inflame the sinuses and lead to congestion and post-nasal drip.

Other symptoms that involve the upper esophagus and airways are bad breath, chronic ear pain, voice change, and vocal cord polyps.

These symptoms can often be elusive and many patients only realize that their cause is GERD after consultation with many doctors. Many patients undergo exhaustive evaluations by specialists other than gastroenterologists, since these symptoms are not commonly thought to be associated with acid reflux disease.

NAUSEA Most patients with reflux do not experience nausea; some do. In those who do experience nausea, one must consider chronic acid exposure. In some patients who experience nausea from reflux, the cause can be an obstruction from a cancer that has formed at the end of the esophagus, severe inflammation (esophagitis), or a benign blockage in the esophagus called a stricture. A stricture can be a result of scar formation in those who experience chronic reflux. Nausea can also be experienced in those who frequently drink alcoholic beverages or take medications that can independently cause nausea.

PERSISTENT COUGH A persistent cough is a very common occurrence in those with reflux disease. The most common causes of a chronic cough are asthma, post-nasal drip, respiratory tract infections, and smoking. Chronic cough is often caused by acid reflux. If patients with a chronic cough have not responded to antibiotics, or other specialists have ruled out other causes, the diagnosis of GERD should be considered, particularly in non-smoking patients.

THROAT OR ESOPHAGUS PAIN Throat pain can mean many different things to different people. It can mean that there is discomfort, burning or pressure underneath the xyphoid (a small bone in the middle of your chest just above your abdomen) which can be a result of acid reflux alone. It can also be esophagitis (inflammation) or worse yet, ulcers at the end of the esophagus. To others, it can be a feeling of food getting stuck in the esophagus (dysphagia) which can last hours if there is a food impaction.
These dysphagia symptoms are generally caused by the presence of scar tissue that has formed in reaction to chronic acid reflux. The scar tissue often forms in rings, called Schatzki's rings or reflux strictures. Less frequently, dysphagia is caused by actual cancers that have formed a narrowing and partial blockage of the passage through the esophagus. These patients often experience pain or produce excess saliva. Some-

times, in patients with dysphagia, food becomes trapped or impacted in the esophagus. This condition usually causes discomfort, and often pain. Occasionally, food becomes so impacted that an ulcer forms in the already inflamed esophagus. This condition may lead to worsening symptoms and the need for surgery. Without a resolution of symptoms, the patient should immediately seek the assistance of a gastroenterologist. If the food is not cleared, the esophagus can be badly injured.

Others experience throat pain because the acid can reflux as high as the pharynx (throat) or larynx (voicebox). This can cause inflammation anywhere along the esophagus, airways, or even up into the mouth.

Throat pain therefore, is rather non-specific, and if due to GERD, may also suggest a variety of problems depending upon the degree of irritation and reflux.

## Other Symptoms

Other symptoms associated with acid reflux include excessive belching, upset stomach, night sweats, awakening during the night choking or coughing or pain, excess salivation (with occasional soilage of a pillow) chronic sinus infections, gingivitis, dental enamel loss, chest pressure, and halitosis (bad breath).

Certain sexual practices have also been identified as a cause of reflux symptoms. A study of 100 women with chronic GERD found that 77 complained of worsening reflux during intercourse. One contributing factor appeared to be coitus performed in the conventional horizontal position (missionary position), which may place too much pressure on the woman's chest.

## "Alarm" Symptoms

The most important alarm symptom is also the most common and elusive one: heartburn. Patients who have experienced heartburn for many years often treat themselves inadequately, just enough to rid themselves of extreme symptoms. They may allow mild reflux to occur chronically, and may even become dependent on daily or multi-weekly over-the-counter antacid therapies. While they may have successfully eliminated at least some of the symptoms of acid reflux, these patients may have caused damage to the esophagus. Remember: Up to 13 percent of the adult population experiences reflux more than twice a week. Other "alarm" symptoms in reflux patients include vomiting blood, dysphagia (the feeling of having something caught in the esophagus), weight loss, excess fatigue, and painful swallowing.

How common are these symptoms? Because GERD is one of the most common of all diseases, its symptoms are also very common. Symptoms are the body's warning signs that something is amiss. No matter how common they are, those symptoms should be taken seriously, particularly if they persist or seem to be different than usual.

When do symptoms usually occur? Sometimes symptoms occur very quickly. If you gulp down a carbonated beverage faster than you should, you may feel the effects almost immediately. More than half of the people I see report that their reflux symptoms almost always occur after eating, particularly after eating fatty meals, spicy foods, alcohol, or chocolate.

Other times, symptoms may not occur until hours after eating or drinking. In fact, about 10 percent of patients experience nighttime heartburn. This typically occurs a few hours after reclining after a late meal or snack. Many patients report that symptoms usually occur when they're asleep, and that those symptoms often awaken them in the middle of the night. This is an interesting finding because our studies indicate that most acid reflux actually occurs during the day, shortly after eating. The mechanism for acid reflux during sleep takes the following course: The LES relaxation occurs naturally after eating when the sphincter opens up allowing food to pass into the stomach. That gives the reflux time to occur whether you eat during the day or just before you go to sleep.

Other patients may have transient relaxation of the lower esophageal sphincter occurring sporadically at odd times during the day followed by acid reflux.

Since digestion is a continuous process, almost everyone experiences these symptoms at one time or another; in fact, 30 to 40 percent of all Americans have symptoms at least once a month. Sometimes symptoms go away in a few minutes or last only for as long as it takes an antacid to neutralize the acid that causes the symptom.

In other instances, however, no matter what the person does, the symptoms either recur intermittently and frequently, last for several hours, occur in stressful situations or occur after nearly every meal. Symptoms that are very intense, very frequent or very persistent are danger signs—your body's way of telling you that you definitely need to seek medical help.

Are the symptoms of GERD easily confused with the symptoms of other diseases? Yes. And that's why it is important to pay particular attention to any symptoms that seem in any way out of the ordinary to you. GERD can be difficult to diagnose, particularly because of the varying ways that it presents itself. For example, what sometimes feels like heartburn is a heart attack. Similarly, persistent pain or irritation in the throat may well be GERD, but it may also be a warning sign of cancer.

Because there are so many medications and advertisements for herbal and alternative treatments on the market today, it is often very difficult to know what to do. While it certainly is possible to try them until you find something that seems to work, it is wiser to consult your doctor to find out what your body is really trying to tell you. These symptoms, as unpleasant as they may be, are your first line of defense against further complications from GERD.

FOOTNOTES
1. Kirk, AJ: Reflux Dyspareunia. Thorax 1986;41:215-216.

# 4

# SEEING A DOCTOR
## *Helping Your Physician Help You*

I F YOU HAVE ANY OF THE "ALARM" SYMPTOMS
mentioned in Chapter III, you should certainly see a doctor.
Frequently, patients with "alarm" symptoms take over-the-
counter (OTC) antacids on a regular basis and can't seem to
live without them. These patients may take them for years and, because
they have become accustomed to the routine, may actually forget that
they have a problem. If these patients stop these medicines, the result
is reflux. Dependency on OTC medicines definitely warrants a medical evaluation.

Other alarm symptoms that require immediate medical evaluation
are the vomiting up of blood, dysphagia (a feeling that food is getting
stuck in the esophagus), odynophagia (pain with swallowing food),
weight loss, and excess fatigue. Patients with chronic reflux symptoms
who also experience weight loss and fatigue should seek a thorough
evaluation, particularly to rule out cancer or other serious causes for
such symptoms.

## *What Kind of Doctor Should You See?*

Because GERD is such a common illness, your family physician has
probably seen many patients who have it. In many cases, he or she

will be able to either recommend non-prescription medications or prescribe a medication for you. You might also expect that your family doctor will recommend a few lifestyle changes like more exercise or a different diet.

If, however, you do not respond to the recommendations made by your family doctor, he or she may suggest that you see a specialist, probably a gastroenterologist, a doctor who is expert in all of the organs that comprise your digestive system. These include the esophagus, stomach, small and large intestine (including the rectum), liver, pancreas, bile ducts, and the gallbladder. All gastroenterologists are trained to treat reflux and other acid related illnesses as well as all types of digestive tract diseases. There are no separate board exams for different categories of gastroenterologists. Any board certified gastroenterologist is highly trained to diagnose and recognize GERD and will be able to treat you with the appropriate lifestyle and medical treatments.

Some gastroenterologists, those who are interested only in diseases of the esophagus, will primarily see patients with esophageal ailments. If you find yourself seeing multiple doctors without clear-cut answers, you may want to consider going to a center that has expertise in this area. Once you get to a qualified gastroenterologist, you should expect to be evaluated and treated thoroughly.

Those people with "alarm" symptoms should certainly notify their family or general doctor, who will in all likelihood refer them directly to a gastroenterologist for further evaluation.

## Preparing for a Gastroenterology Appointment

Specialists like gastroenterologists are to the medical profession what detectives are to the police department. Their job is to take what is known about your situation and find a solution to the problem. Like a police detective, they start by gathering as much information as possible. The first step in this process is for you to compile your own information. Although it may seem to you that some of the information your doctor wants has no relevance to your situation, just as in a police investigation, sometimes the smallest, or what seems like the most insignificant clue can be the one that solves the case.

The best gastroenterologists are those who will spend time listening to you describe your symptoms. Some questions that a gastroenterologist may ask are questions about your family history, sexual history, childhood history, and eating and drinking habits. Other questions may be related to issues such as psychosocial stressors and relationships. Patients with such problems may have altered sleep cycles, patterns of caffeine and drug intake, as well as other factors that can provoke symptoms. When asked these questions patients often say, "Why are you asking me that question? It has nothing to do with my reflux?!" Answers to these general questions may help to give the physician extra insight into the patient's condition and influence the outcome of the disease.

Since lifestyle modifications are key, you should expect a good doctor to delve into the above issues with you. You should never be embarrassed about what is revealed in these discussions. Whatever you discuss with your doctor remains confidential. Your doctor is not there to make value judgments about you, only to help you treat your disease. And in order to do that effectively, the doctor must understand all the factors that might be contributing to it.

WHAT SHOULD YOU BRING TO THE DOCTOR'S OFFICE? Whether you are visiting your family doctor or a specialist such as a gastroenterologist, it is very helpful if you bring along the following items:

Food Diary. GERD is a disease of the digestive tract, so to determine what has caused your discomfort, your doctor will need to know precisely what you are accustomed to eating and drinking. Therefore, it is very important that for at least a week prior to your appointment you keep a detailed food diary. In it, you should list:

1. *What* you eat and drink
2. *How much* of each thing you eat and drink
3. *Exactly when* you eat and drink them
4. *Where* you eat and drink them
5. *What you do following* eating and drinking

It is also helpful to list symptoms that you experience and when you experience them in relation to your food intake. This may help the doctor correlate your symptoms with the specific foods that you are eating. Below is a sample of what your food diary for one day might look like:

**DATE:** May 1

| Food/Beverage | Quantity | Time | Place | Activity | Symptom ? |
|---|---|---|---|---|---|
| Reg. Coffee | 3 cups | 7 A.M. | Home | Leave for work | |
| Half & Half | 3 tsps | Same | Same | Same | |
| Sugar | 3 tsps | Same | Same | Same | |
| White toast | 1 slice | Same | Same | Same | |
| Grape Jelly | 1 tbl. | Same | Same | Same | |
| Fried eggs | 2 | Same | Same | Same | |
| Bacon | 2 strips | Same | Same | Same | 8 A.M.: Acid in chest |
| Glazed donut | 1 | 10 A.M. | Work | Continue work | |
| Regular Coke | 1 can | Same | Same | Same | |
| Cheeseburger | 1 | Noon | Café | Back to work | |
| French fries | 1 small | Same | Same | Same | |
| Regular Coffee | 2 cups | Same | Same | Same | |
| Instant creamer | 2 pkgs | Same | Same | Same | |
| Sugar | 2 pkgs | Same | Same | Same | |
| Peppermint | 1 | Same | Same | Same | 12:30 P.M.: Bad chest pain; lasted 30min. |
| Regular Coke | 1 bottle | 3:00 P.M. | Same | Same | |
| Beer | 1 bottle | 6:00 P.M. | Home | Watch TV | |
| Pork Chop | 1 (6oz.) | 6:30 P.M. | Same | Same | |
| Green beans | 1 cup | Same | Same | Same | |
| Butter | 1 tsp | Same | Same | Same | |
| Mashed potatoes | 1 cup | Same | Same | Same | |
| Gravy | 1/2 cup | Same | Same | Same | |
| Vanilla ice cream | 1 cup | 10 P.M. | Same | Go to bed | Midnight: Awakened, fire in chest |

Notice that everything, including the after-lunch peppermint, was included in this food diary, because even the smallest item can cause a problem.

**A List of All Medications You Take.** As does your food diary, this list needs to be very complete. Many people forget about some of the medicines they take or don't include vitamin supplements and herbal supplements, which are medications, as well. Since you have limited time with your doctor, it's important that you remember your medicines and preferably either bring them in or bring a list with you. It's a major factor in GERD. Your list should include:

1.  All *prescription medications* you take
2.  All *non-prescription medications* you take
3.  All *vitamin supplements* you take
4.  All *herbal medications* you take
5.  All *food supplements* you take

As with your food diary, you should also list the exact quantity you take, when you take it, where you take it and what you do following the time you take it. Below is a sample medication list.

**DATE:** May 1

| MEDICATION | QUANTITY | TIME | PLACE | ACTIVITY FOLLOWING |
|---|---|---|---|---|
| Safeway Aspirin | 1 | 6 A.M. | Home | Eat breakfast |
| Lipitor | 1 (20MG) | 6 A.M. | Same | Same |
| Vioxx | 1 (25MG) | 6 A.M. | Same | Same |
| Nature Made Vitamin E | 1 (400 I.U.) | 7 A.M. | Same | Go to work |
| Member's Mark Vitamin C | 1 (500MG) | 7 A.M. | Same | Same |
| Shaklee Alfalfa Tab | 1 TABLET | 7 A.M. | Same | Same |
| Tums | 2 TABLETS | 10 A.M. | Work | Go back to work |
| Tylenol | 2 (500MG) | 3 P.M. | Same | Go back to work |
| Tums | 2 TABLETS | 8:30 P.M. | Home | Watch TV |

**Lifestyle Diary.** Because GERD may also be caused by certain lifestyle choices, it is also very helpful to your doctor if you bring to your appointment a diary of what a week's worth of normal activity for you would look like. Below is a sample.

**DATE:** May 1

| ACTIVITY | DURATION OF ACTIVITY | TIME | LOCATION | FOLLOWING ACTIVITY |
|---|---|---|---|---|
| Get up | | 5:45 A.M. | Home | Go to work |
| Arrive at work | | 8 A.M. | Office | Go to lunch |
| Lunch | 1 hour | 12–1 P.M. | Restaurant | Go back to work |
| Leave work | | 5:00 P.M. | Go home | |
| Play Racquetball | 2 hours | 8–10 P.M. | Gym at work | Go home |

**WHAT WILL THE DOCTOR ASK YOU?** Before you see the doctor, you'll be asked to fill out a detailed medical questionnaire. You'll need to provide the following information:

1. *Date*
2. *Identifying data* about you (age, sex, race, place of birth, marital status, occupation and so on)
3. A *detailed family history* of your blood relatives
4. If you have been *referred by another doctor*, as well as the names and addresses of that doctor or other doctors who have treated you
5. What *present illnesses or complaints* you may have (Usually in the form of a checklist.)
6. What *illnesses or complaints you have had in the past* (Sometimes this is part of the same checklist as your past medical history.)
7. A *review history* asking if you've had problems with any of your other bodily systems, such as urinary tract, lungs, skin, heart and other organs
8. What *medications* you are now taking. If you can attach the medication diary described below it will be very helpful.
9. What, if anything, you are *allergic* to
10. *Whether you smoke or drink alcohol* and, if so, how much
11. Whether you take any *narcotic drugs*

12. A *detailed social history* including a relationship history.
13. A *psychiatric history*
14. The *time you last had diagnostic tests* such as a tuberculin test, pap smear, mammogram, cholesterol check, prostate check and a test for anemia.
15. Whether you have received treatment for *mental illness*.
16. *Previous x-rays* including upper GI series, upper endoscopy, barium studies, small bowel series, sonogram of abdomen/liver or gallbladder, and esophageal motility studies (also known as manometry studies). *(We'll discuss these tests in chapter 5.)*

## The Doctor–Patient Interaction

The medical interview will allow you to openly discuss your history (past and current) with the doctor. He or she will ask a multitude of questions and will often direct the conversation in a manner that best identifies potential problems.

Most patients prefer not to disclose personal information in front of family members or friends. If you strongly wish to have a family member present, you should be prepared to answer even personal questions with them in the room; otherwise, you may want to ask them to stay in the waiting room.

Parents of younger patients often come with the expectation that they will be in the room speaking and listening the entire time. Most parents want to speak for their children (because they are concerned) and it becomes very difficult for the patient to speak about habits such as drugs, alcohol, sexual history, and eating habits. For these reasons family members are asked to wait in the waiting area.

A physical examination is performed. Patients are told what is being examined and why. After the examination there is a review of the findings. If it is possible, the patient is told whether there is a normal or abnormal finding.

## The Physical Examination

The physical examination performed by your gastroenterologist is typically a focused examination of your digestive organs, however certain other areas are often examined, too, depending on the history you give. After this, a detailed gastrointestinal exam will follow.

The abdominal examination usually starts with listening to your abdomen to elicit bowel sound activity. After this, the doctor will place his/her hands over your abdomen and will likely press firmly to feel for your organs and to elicit abnormalities. You may feel some mild discomfort from the pressure.

The last part of the exam is often the rectal exam, in which a gloved finger is placed into your anus. This is a very useful examination as it can detect the presence of microscopic blood in the stool that you may not be able to see in the toilet bowl or with your eyes. This exam is very important, particularly if you have symptoms of abdominal or chest pain or if you have a known anemia. A rectal exam usually lasts only a few seconds and most say that the anticipation and fear of the exam is actually much worse than the exam itself.

## Wrap-Up Discussion

After the examination, the doctor will discuss with the patient anything he or she has found, as well as a diagnostic plan and/or any test recommendations. The wrap-up is intended to be a summation of the findings. After this portion of the consultation, the patient will either be sent to the laboratory for blood work, or to a secretary to schedule various tests.

After the evaluation, if a work-up is indicated, a long term plan with both a diagnosis and a treatment plan are initiated. Many GERD patients may see their physicians at least twice a year. Some see them more frequently depending on the severity of symptoms. At each office visit, findings are typically communicated with the referral physician in the form of updates. In these letters, a report reviewing all of the gastroenterologist's findings are sent to the referring physician, as well as the results of any tests the specialist ordered for the patient. Once the patient's symptoms are under control, and no further treatment is necessary, the specialist advises both the patient and referring doctor that his treatment has been completed. At this point, the family doctor will often take over general care of the patient based on the gastroenterologist's recommendations. Patients with milder disease or symptoms can typically be followed by their general physician. In the more complicated cases, the specialist may have to follow the patient long-term.

## Diagnostic Testing and Continued Visits to the Specialist

After the doctor has studied your medical history (including the diaries you have completed), reviewed all findings, and made a plan for you, he or she may suggest that you undergo some diagnostic tests. These tests are described in the following chapter. If your physician feels that further tests are not necessary, the physician may go ahead and prescribe a medicine for you to take. A follow-up appointment is usually scheduled in the near future to review your condition.

# 5

# Diagnosing GERD
## *What to Expect*

THE FIRST STEP IN CONDUCTING A MEDICAL investigation is to get as much information as possible. The second step is to conduct one or more tests to learn even more about the patient's discomfort. Based on the information a patient supplies and additional information derived from medical tests, physicians, like detectives, can "solve the case" and offer the patient a specific diagnosis based on the symptoms and the test results.

A diagnosis is achieved by following one or more of the following diagnostic procedures:

### *Direct Conversation*

Although your doctor will carefully study the written information you have provided, he or she will also want to spend time talking with you directly. Direct conversation builds on the information gained from written documents like questionnaires and diaries and helps the doctor understand the less tangible nature of your distress. For example, the doctor will likely ask you to describe not just what is bothering you, but how often you experience discomfort and how severe it is.

Before you see your family doctor or a specialist, such as a gastroenterologist, it is important that you anticipate three important questions that will likely be asked of you.

1. What is the *quality* of your pain (i.e. mild, moderate or severe)?
2. What is the *character* of your pain (i.e. sharp, dull, dagger-like, achy, etc.)?
3. What is the *duration* of your pain (seconds, minutes, hours)?

Patients often have a hard time grading pain. They often say they "have trouble describing it" or tell the doctor they will pay more attention to it before the next visit. Since the best time to accurately describe pain is when you are in the doctor's office, thinking about questions like pain grading in advance greatly helps the doctor diagnose your disease.

## *Direct Observation*

After the doctor has discussed your written information with you and talked with you about symptoms your are experiencing, like pain, he or she will conduct an examination of your mouth and the portion of your throat that can be seen externally. Your physician will also note physical conditions that are known to be related to GERD such as:

obesity

anorexia

cancer of the mouth, throat, stomach, or small or (less likely) large intestine.

## Diagnostic Tests

Because GERD is a disease involving internal organs, it is likely your doctor will also conduct or send you to a testing laboratory for one of several diagnostic tests. Some of these tests will pinpoint exactly what it is that is causing your discomfort. Other tests will be conducted to rule out other causes of your symptoms.

Tests that are designed to pinpoint specific causes of GERD include:

**Endoscopy.** Only a small portion of the throat can be seem externally and that portion is often not affected by reflux disease. The entire esophagus, therefore, needs to be examined in patients with chronic disease or patients for whom medicines do not appear to greatly improve symptoms. The most common diagnostic test used to examine the esophagus is called an upper endoscopy (EGD). It is important to note that most patients with GERD do not need this procedure. Only those with chronic disease (usually more than 4 to 5 years of reflux) or refractory disease (those patients whose symptoms do not improve completely with antacids) should consider an upper endoscopy evaluation.

For this procedure, some doctors will first anesthetize the throat with a local anesthetic. Most doctors use cetacaine in the form of a spray or a swab. Administering this anesthetic is painless and the effects of the anesthetic wear off in 30 to 60 minutes. In the United States, most gastroenterologists also have the option of using intravenous medicines to sedate patients if they prefer or if other factors make this a more desirable choice.

If IV sedation is used, a nurse will place an intravenous line into a vein in the arm and then inject a sedative into the line. Demerol (meperidine) and Versed (midazolam) are commonly used combinations for intravenous sedation although some facilities use other drugs that have similar effects. These drugs are given just before the procedure and are used to reduce pain and anxiety.

Some doctors do not use these medicines in testing patients who are very ill or at high risk for sedatives. In some cases, doctors may even do the procedure without sedation. The procedure is short and the tube is narrow, so it can certainly be done safely without sedation, however, it may be somewhat uncomfortable.

If you are concerned about taking a sedative, you may want to ask your doctor about the type of sedation that will be used. There are also certain potential side effects that patients should be informed of prior to consenting to the procedure. In the vast majority of cases, the patient awakens comfortable and pain free, although occasionally, there is a mild sore throat after the procedure which can last a few days.

Once the throat is anesthetized, the doctor will insert an endoscope down your throat and through your esophagus. In patients with GERD although the esophagus is the most important place to look for damage, most doctors will also include an evaluation of your entire stomach as well as the beginning of the small intestine (the duodenum). Evaluating these areas will ensure that your symptoms are not ulcer related. If they are ulcer related, they may require more directed therapy.

The endoscope is a slender tube with a light and tiny camera attached to a machine that is able to magnify the images from inside your body and project them onto a large TV screen. This instrument allows the doctor to thoroughly examine the surface of the esophagus without using surgery.

During this procedure the doctor looks for the following signs: inflammation (esophagitis); ulcers in the esophagus, stomach or duodenum; cancers; scar tissue (called strictures) or a condition known as Barrett's esophagus. Barrett's causes a change in the appearance of the esophagus that results from chronic acid reflux injury. Looking for signs of Barrett's esophagus is very important because it is considered a precancerous condition.

Because the endoscope diameter is so narrow, this procedure is very safe and patients seldom experience any aftereffects. The entire procedure is typically complete in a half hour and patients often wake up wondering when the procedure will begin!

It is important to recognize that some patients may have GERD with symptoms, but have no visible changes to the lining of the esophagus seen during an endoscopy. If the endoscopic procedure reveals nothing abnormal about your esophagus or that no overt signs of damage are present, the doctor may suggest another very sensitive test called a pH probe.

pH PROBE. Because GERD always involves stomach acid, and since an endoscopic examination may reveal little or no damage, an important part of diagnosis is assessing just how much acid is refluxing into the esophagus. Reflux is a chronic problem, so to get a clear picture of both the recurrence and severity of the problem, it is helpful if the doctor can determine whether there is acid in the esophagus and if there is, when and where it occurs.

In most patients, the length of the esophagus is 35 to 40 centimeters from the two front teeth to the stomach. Most GERD patients who also have associated esophageal damage, have it in the last one-third to one-fourth of the esophagus. The pH study allows the gastroenterologist to assess whether there is acid anywhere along the entire length of the esophagus.

The pH probe, like an endoscope, is a very fine tube; however, unlike the endoscope, it is a measuring device, rather than a visual device. It is inserted into the nose and threaded down the esophagus to the lower esophageal sphincter.

The pH probe measures the pH (the degree of alkalinity or acidity) present in the esophagus and records this information on a box the patient wears on a belt around the waist. It is usually in place for 24 hours, during which time the patient is asked to eat and drink normally so the probe can gauge when the greatest discomfort seems to occur.

Although the probe can cause temporary irritation and discomfort, it produces few, if any, aftereffects. The probe allows the doctor to correlate symptoms and document them on a time sheet with actual measurements of acid in the esophagus. It greatly helps to differentiate reflux discomfort from non-reflux causes of pain. When having this test, it is important not to take any acid preparations (over-the-counter or prescription) five to seven days before the procedure.

ESOPHAGEAL MANOMETRY. In addition to measuring the amount of acid reflux present, the doctor may also measure the amount of pressure within the esophagus and lower esophagael sphincter. The test is called manometry. Patients who are referred for it are typically those in whom the upper endoscopy and pH studies reveal normal or equivocal (ambiguous) results.

This test allows the doctor to analyze the muscular activity of the esophagus and assess whether there is appropriate timing of the contractions. It can also identify those patients with abnormal peristalsis. Patients with chest pain or discomfort may have a problem with the muscles of the esophagus. A manometry study is the best way to measure the efficiency of the peristaltic motion of the esophagus.

Measuring pressure involves the use of a thin tube that is inserted through the nose and passed into the esophagus. A lubricant is used to allow for passage of the tube, but no sedatives are required. The patient helps by swallowing while the instrument is inserted. The tube is passed down the esophagus to the lower esophagael sphincter.

The patient is asked to take a series of dry swallows (swallowing only saliva) and wet swallows (with water) repeatedly throughout the test to aid in obtaining various pressure measurements at various intervals in the esophagus. At this point, the measurements are made to evaluate strength and normalcy of the peristalsic contractions. Some patients have abnormally high contractions in the esophagus that can cause pain. Others may have poor contractions that may make reflux worse because the esophagus can no longer clear acid by use of contractile activity. The prolonged acid exposure that results can also lead to damage and injury, or at least, discomfort. The manometry study can easily detect patients who have a problem with decreased lower esophageal sphincter pressure, a common cause of reflux.

Some tests are designed to rule out other causes for GERD symptoms. These include:

ELECTROCARDIOGRAM (ECG). Because chest pain is one of the most common symptoms of GERD, the doctor may want you to have an electrocardiogram. This test is frequently used in the emergency room as a quick test for chest pain, but your gastroenterologist may also request that you have one. For this test, several sensors are attached to your chest, arms and legs. These sensors are small rubber disks that are attached to tubes that are connected to an electrocardiograph machine. The electrocardiograph records the electrical activity that occurs during each heartbeat and can help the doctor determine any abnormalities or disease of the heart. The test is completely painless, takes only a few minutes and requires no anesthetic. Generally, the doctor can give the results of the electrocardiogram test immediately after the test is complete. Obviously, the most important reason to have this test is to rule out the possibility of a heart attack or any other cardiac irregularities.

X-RAY. General X-rays are often performed in those who have excessive bloating or distention. They have little role in the workup of GERD. However, if the doctor suspects another cause for your discomfort, such as a bowel obstruction (particularly if you have had surgery in the past), an abdominal X-ray may be warranted.

BARIUM ESOPHAGRAM. This important test is often the first one ordered by the doctor, even before an endoscopy. It is non-invasive and takes little time. The radiologist has the patient swallow a white chalky material called barium, after which X-rays of the chest are taken. The X-rays can show blockages in the esophagus, narrowing, and other anatomic abnormalities. In some cases the X-rays can also reveal reflux.

VIDEO-ESOPHAGRAM. Like a barium esophagram, a video-esophagram evaluates the esophagus via X-ray. This test, however, will be a live video X-ray of the chest while you swallow liquid or solid food. This test allows the radiologist to examine the swallowing mechanism of your upper throat and esophagus muscles. It can identify patients with poor muscle activity that results in aspiration of material into the lungs and allows the radiologist to see, on video, reflux of swallowed material back into the esophagus or even into the lungs. Like a barium esophagram, a video-esophagram can identify blockages in the esophagus, as well. This test is a preferred test for those who are being evaluated for reflux but have not yet had an upper endoscopy, or do not wish to have one. The only problem with this test is that it can miss the finding of esophagitis or ulcers in the esophagus.

## Making the Diagnosis

FUNCTIONAL DISORDERS. One of the most challenging things about making a specific diagnosis of GERD is that, despite the fact that it is so common, it can often be very difficult to pin down to a specific cause. Some patients experience a great deal of chest pain. Others have bloating, acid indigestion or belching. Yet, even after conducting the most sophisticated tests, there is little physical evidence that anything is wrong. When this is the case, the doctor may suggest a "functional disorder," that is, something that is very real to you, but cannot be found by the tests.

There are other tests, such as a gastric emptying study, which are able to detect functional disorders. If they are negative as well, the diagnosis is often made by a "diagnosis of exclusion," which means that since all objective tests have been negative, then a functional disorder is likely to be responsible. These disorders are often difficult to treat, but there are options.

Such cases can be extremely frustrating to patients who may have been told by a variety of doctors that their disease must be a psychological problem rather than a physical one. By contrast, other patients come with only minor symptoms and yet the tests reveal that they have sustained a large amount of physical damage.

RULING OUT OTHER CAUSES. Often, the first thing we do in making a diagnosis, is identifying what the disease is not. One of these we must rule out, certainly, is heart disease. Generally, we can do this by finding out whether or not the symptoms are relieved by antacids. Antacids will often relieve GERD symptoms, but seldom those of heart disease. If the patient reveals that sitting up while drinking or eating, avoiding late night or fatty meals, and avoiding "reflux foods" tends to lessen symptoms, this also strongly supports the diagnosis of reflux.

Using the tests described earlier, we can also rule out other serious diseases such as cancer, and a variety of musculoskeletal or rheumatologic disorders such as scleroderma or achalasia (to be discussed later). Although, sometimes GERD may be the result of several different things occurring at the same time, so we must also take this into consideration.

Whatever the cause or causes, however, it is important for your doctor to work closely with you to develop a diagnosis that pinpoints the cause of your discomfort. Only then can an effective course of treatment be recommended.

# 6

# CAUSES OF GERD
## *Food, Lifestyle Choices & More*

G ASTROESOPHAGEAL REFLUX DISEASE CAN result from a variety of "insults" that interfere with the systems that clear acid from the esophagus. Normally, acid does not reflux into the esophagus to a great degree. In GERD patients, however, the protective and precise mechanics of esophageal clearance are disturbed to the point that symptoms are present. Although there are many technical medical terms for the causes of GERD, generally speaking, its is caused by one or a combination of five factors:

1.  *Lifestyle choices*
2.  *Reaction to foods or beverages*
3.  *Reaction to medication*
4.  *Systemic diseases,* conditions or injury to the upper GI tract
5.  *Congenital malformation or abnormality* of the esophago-gastric digestive system.
6.  *Occupational hazards*

Although everyone may be able to tolerate small physiologic amounts of reflux without any significant symptoms, a combination of adverse factors can lead not only to the discomfort of heartburn but to injury of the esophagus as well.

## Lifestyle Choices

**SMOKING.** Smoking is the leading preventable cause of death in the United States. While the negative effects of smoking are most commonly associated with respiratory problems, such as asthma, smoking may even harm babies born to mothers who smoke during pregnancy. Smoking has also been shown to be a major factor in the development of cancers of the lung, pancreas, bladder, mouth, tongue, oropharynx, larynx, cervix, and esophagus. Because cancer in the esophagus can cause considerable scarring, inflammation, and destruction of the normal smooth esophageal lining, those who have it can experience great difficulty in swallowing. Difficulty swallowing is a major cause of GERD in these patients, because the precise muscle and nerve impulses of the esophagus are inhibited by the cancer and its local effects. Cancer also causes abnormalities in peristalic contractions as well as in the clearance mechanisms that expel secretions that are normally made by the mouth and esophagus to protect the esophagus from injury.

**ALCOHOL INTAKE.** Alcohol is the most commonly overused drug in our society. In addition to damaging the heart, liver, brain, and reproductive organs, excessive alcohol use can cause acute gastritis in the stomach and is a main causative agent in cancer of the mouth, throat, larynx, tongue, lips, and esophagus. Alcohol can directly harm the esophagus by reducing the lower esophageal sphincter (LES) pressure and increasing the gastric acid exposure to the esophagus. As a direct irritant, it can also make esophagitis from heartburn worse by its toxic effect on the esophageal lining, and it can make symptomatic heartburn even worse.

**STRESS.** There is no scientific data to support the theory that stress is a direct cause of GERD. One complication is that stress is often difficult to measure objectively. Some individuals thrive on a fast-paced lifestyle, eat on the run, stay up until all hours of the night, and seem to experience few digestive problems. Other people experience severe discomfort if there is the slightest deviation from their normal routine.

GERD, however, can cause a great deal of stress and anxiety, since the condition can be severe and quite symptomatic. Although stress may not be directly implicated, in some patients it has been shown to contribute to a sensation that the throat is closing up (globus sensation) as well as a feeling of chest tightness, palpitations, and shortness of breath. In patients with these symptoms, reflux is often found to occur.

CLOTHING. Patients prone to GERD, often experience worsening symptoms when they wear tight-fitting clothing that creates pressure on the stomach. The effect is purely a pressure phenomenon: The more pressure on the stomach, the more acid will reflux into the esophagus.

SEDENTARY LIFESTYLE. Although vigorous exercise can cause acid reflux, a sedentary lifestyle can also promote GERD. Those who are sedentary are at a greater risk for weight gain and poor diets consisting of foods that may reduce the lower esophageal sphincter pressure. Patients with sedentary lifestyles are not only at risk for GERD, but are also at risk for many other health problems, as well, including overweight and its related issues.

EATING CLOSE TO BEDTIME. Late dinners are commonplace in many households. When people consume their last, and often heaviest, meal the stomach distends with food, causing the LES to expand and stretch. If this is compounded by intake of foods that stimulate reflux (fatty foods, alcohol, caffeine) the LES tone is further reduced. When the patient reclines shortly after the meal, gastric acid reflux is further enhanced by gravity.

SLEEPING ON A FLAT BED. The majority of people who experience reflux do so during the daytime—primarily after meals. Those who experience severe nighttime reflux can often be awakened with burning and pain. For those who are prone to reflux, a flat surface alone can induce or worsen symptoms, even if the meal was eaten three or more hours before bedtime.

## Reaction to Foods or Beverages

HIGH FAT DIET. Advocates of the popular Atkins diet contend that a high fat diet is healthy. However, many physicians argue that a diet high in fat is unhealthy for a number of reasons. High fat diets can contribute to weight gain, obesity, and cardiovascular problems. Fat is also known to be a potent contributor to reflux disease, since a diet high in fat decreases lower esophageal sphincter pressure and increases the likelihood of reflux symptoms in those people prone to reflux.

ACIDIC FOODS. Although stomach acid is 100 times more acidic than acid in foods, foods that have a high acid content can still cause trouble. Acidic foods and spices, although not directly implicated in the cause of acid reflux, are thought to irritate the already erosive surface of the esophagus in those who already have reflux. Since acid is not intended to be in the esophagus, those consuming acidic or spicy foods or beverages can have a sharp increase of reflux from the possible irritation on the esophageal mucosa from such foods.

LARGE PORTIONS. Spices and acidic foods are often blamed for heartburn; however, a greater problem may be eating large portions. Although the stomach's capacity is quite large, it's capacity for food is limited. The acid secreted by the stomach lining can act only so fast. Gastric acid is released in response to food to aid digestion in the stomach. But when the LES is weakened or the expansive forces of the stomach are challenged, the food and the gastric acid may reflux into the esophagus. The prolonged contact of gastric acid on esophageal mucosa then becomes the factor responsible for esophageal irritation with secondary pain. If the reflux persists or is chronic, esophageal ulceration may result.

Once the stomach is full of food, the normal course it takes is downward into the small intestine for digestion and reflux does not occur. If the food is forced back up into the esophagus, the result is GERD.

## Reactions to Medication

There are a variety of medicines that may contribute to GERD. Because some medications may make your symptoms worse, if you have GERD, you should ask your doctor whether or not you need to remain on these medications.

Neurologic Medications:
- *Alpha adrenergic antagonists*
- *Anticholinergics*
- *Anti-psychotics*
- *Barbiturates*
- *Beta adrenergic antagonists*

Other Medications and Chemicals:
- *Aspirin*
- *Barbiturates*
- *Calcium channel blockers*
- *Diazepam*
- *Meperidine*
- *Morphine*
- *Nicotine*
- *Nitrates*
- *Non steroidal anti-inflammatory drugs (NSAIDS)*
- *Progesterone (often increased in early pregnancy)*
- *Serotonin*
- *Smooth muscle relaxants*

## Systemic Diseases

Systemic diseases are processes that may affect the human body as a whole, but that may also have profound effects on the esophagus.

These effects can be secondary to involvement in breaking the normal protective barrier of esophageal mucosa. In these cases, the lining of the esophagus is disrupted and damage can result, making the lining more sensitive to gastric acid exposure.

In other cases, the diseases may not involve the integrity of the esophageal lining, but rather may affect the deeper layers of the esophagus, thereby compromising normal peristalic contractions. As peristaltic activity decreases, esophageal clearance of acid also decreases and the esophagus suffers prolonged exposure to acid. That, in turn, increases the likelihood of esophageal injury.

Other diseases can affect the lower esophageal sphincter alone. In such cases, the lining and muscular lining of the esophagus is not compromised. However, the valvelike effect of the LES is disrupted, thereby increasing and enhancing gastro-esophageal reflux.

SCLERODERMA. Scleroderma is a progressive disease that causes the fibrous connective tissue in the skin and internal organs to become inflamed around tiny blood vessels called capillaries. Over time this inflammation causes scarring and as a result the tissues shrink and become stiff. Schleroderma can affect many of the body's organs, but the skin and esophagus are nearly always affected. As the esophagus stiffens, swallowing can become very difficult. Poor esophageal clearance of acid results. The failure of the muscles to contract in the lower esophagus weakens the LES.

Classic symptoms are heartburn (which can be mild to severe) and dysphagia (the sensation of food getting stuck in the esophagus). Severe scars, called strictures, may form in the esophagus in these patients, leading to even more complications.

DIABETES. Diabetes is a disorder in which the pancreas either produce not enough or no insulin at all or in which the body is insensitive to the insulin that the pancreas does produce. As a result, the body does not absorb glucose properly and cells don't receive the nutrients they need to give the body energy. If untreated, diabetes can cause a wide variety of serious problems such as blindness, limb loss, stroke, high blood pressure, and even death. People with diabetes also often suffer from GERD. Although the cause is not clearly understood, diabetes patients who have a condition known as neuropathy have a nearly 60 percent chance of having abnormal peristalsis in the esophagus. It is unclear if this is primarily an effect of diabetes on the neurologic inervation of the esophageal muscles or if there is a direct effect on the muscles of the esophagus. It is generally accepted that diabetes, by affecting the nerves that stimulate muscle contraction, can contribute to GERD.

ASTHMA. The relationship between asthma and GERD is not well understood; however, some 70 to 80 percent of patients with asthma also have GERD. Asthma is a chronic condition that generally affects breathing. It manifests itself typically as wheezing, which may be audible only with a stethoscope. Patients may often feel short of breath.

Many patients with asthma have also been found to have esophageal reflux through a pH monitoring study (a probe worn for 24 hours that measures the acid content of the esophagus). The presumed cause of asthma in such patients is that they intermittently aspirate small quantities of gastric contents into the lungs, secondary to reflux.

Another potential cause of asthma is a reflux mechanism by the vagus nerve, which may be stimulated in those with acid reflux, thereby stimulating the bronchial tissue to constrict.

Patients with asthma may have associated acid reflux and this causative factor should always be considered since anti-reflux medicines often improve or remove the symptoms of asthma.

OBESITY. Obesity is a disorder in which person weighs at least 20 percent more than his or her ideal weight. By this definition, at least 25% of all Americans are obese and among certain age and ethnic groups, the percentage is as high as 60 percent.

Being even slightly overweight adds significantly to the development of GERD. The presumed cause of reflux in obesity is pressure exherted on the abdominal wall with compression of the stomach causing acid to regurgitate into the esophagus. The pressure placed upon the diaphragm, stomach and gastro-esophageal junction has also been implicated as a cause of reflux, although no adequate studies clearly explain this mechanism.

## Conditions

Several conditions (i.e. health problems or temporary changes in physiology that are not strictly speaking, diseases) can also cause GERD. Among them are:

HIATAL HERNIA. A hernia is a bulge or protrusion of soft tissue that forces its way somewhere it does not belong. Hernias can occur many places in the body, but those that cause particular problems for GERD sufferers are called hiatal hernias. These hernias result when a portion of the stomach forces its way through the diaphragm and into the lower end of the esophagus. This blockage can either prevent food from entering the stomach or cause it to back up into the esophagus. Hiatal hernias occur in people of all ages. The condition can evolve over time and worsen, although most people who have them have small clinically insignificant hernias. Many hernias, incidentally, are found with endoscopy and are associated with no symptoms whatsoever. Others, however, are very symptomatic and can cause severe heartburn, chest pain, gas and bloating. Patients with hiatal hernias are prone to relflux.

COUGHING. Coughing can also be both a cause and an effect of GERD. In fact, GERD is responsible for 20 percent of chronic cough among non-smokers. In non-smoking patients with a chronic cough, acid reflux should be considered.

PHARYNGEAL POUCH. Pharyngeal pouch, a condition found mostly in older men, is a bulge at the back of the throat immediately above the top of the esophagus. Like a hiatal hernia, a pharyngeal pouch interferes with the smooth flow of food and liquids through the digestive tract and may cause difficulty swallowing. These pouches typically occur in areas of weakness in the oropharynx—the part of the pharynx that is below the soft palate and above the epiglottis. In some cases, the pouches can fill with fluid or food. If this occurs, patients may have intermittent aspiration of the pouch contents into the airways, causing cough, asthma, or a feeling that food is stuck in the throat.

PREGNANCY. Pregnant women often experience GERD for the same reason that obese people do: pressure on the abdomen. As the baby grows and more pressure is exherted, GERD can be worsened.

GERD is common in pregnant women. In fact, 40 to 80 percent of pregnant women experience reflux at some time during their pregnancy. In addition to pressure, other factors that contribute to reflux in pregnancy include physiologic changes, including hormonal ones. Because of concern for risk to the fetus, many prescription medicines for acid reduction are not recommended; however, some over-the-counter medications are safe to take during pregnancy. Pregnant women should consult their doctor if they suffer from significant reflux throughout their pregnancies.

PRESENCE OF NASOGASTRIC TUBES. Nasogastric tubes are clear plastic tube inserted through the nose and into the stomach to remove air and digestive juices from the stomach or as a feeding tube. And like cigarette smoke or excessive alcohol, the presence of a nasogastric tube causes continuous irritation to the esophagus. In addition, the tube acts as a barrier to effective gastroesophageal closure. This effect has been suggested to further induce reflux in those receiving nasogastric tube feeding. Generally the removal of the tube corrects the problem. But in cases in which a tube must be in place for a long period of time, other forms of feeding should be considered, such as a surgically or endoscopically placed jejunostomy tube (a feeding tube placed beyond the stomach within the small intestine) to reduce the likelihood of gastric reflux of fed contents through a gastrostomy tube.

DIFFUSE SPASMS OF THE ESOPHAGUS. For reasons that are yet unknown, instead of the normal peristaltic motion in the esophagus some people experience spasms that are a result of simultaneous repetitive contractions of the esophagus. These spasms make swallowing difficult and interfere with the smooth flow of food to the stomach. These spasms can also inhibit normal physiological esophageal clearance and can contribute to heartburn and reflux associated injury. Diagnosis of diffuse spasms of the esophagus is made by a test called an esophageal manometry.

ACHALASIA. Achalasia is the general term for a condition in which the lower esophageal ring of muscle (sphincter) fails to relax. This condiiton is diagnosed by esophageal manometry or an upper GI series. The problem is that the nerves controlling the muscles of the lower end of the esophagus are defective. The ring of muscle, the lower esophageal sphincter (LES) that would ordinarily open to allow the food to leave the esophagus and enter the stomach does not relax, and the food remains in the esophagus. Patients with achalasia also have poor peristalsis in the esophagus with a markedly dilated and boggy esophagus and little to no muscle motion to propel food downward. The result can be a bad taste in the mouth or pain in the chest. Food left in the esophagus can also cause chest infections and poses a danger of food being aspirated into the lungs. Achalasia is often a congenital defect, but it can also be caused (although less likely) by other factors such as disease or injury.

Achalasia occurs in degrees. Some people experience slight achalasia, while others develop severe problems in which the sphincter does not work at all. Patients with this disease should be monitored by a gastroenterologist, as the condition is chronic and progressive. Early intervention is important in order to prevent worsening and irreversible disease. Most patients with achalasia experience reflux symptoms.

## Injury

ESOPHAGEAL CANCER. In cancer of the esophagus, also known as adenocarcinoma, the cells in the lining of the esophagus begin to increase rapidly and form tumors that can spread to other parts of the body. If untreated, the tumors can narrow the esophagus and effectively close off the opening to the stomach. Although it is not known exactly what causes cancer of the esophagus, it is thought that continuous irritation to the esophagus due to smoking, excess alcohol consumption, or GERD may trigger the disease. Because reflux is an irritant, in some people, GERD may be both the cause and the effect of the cancer. Patients with chronic reflux may also be at risk for a condition called "Barret's esophagus" (See Chapter 16). This condition can predispose the patient to esophageal cancer.

It is recommended that patients with chronic reflux, have surveillance upper endoscopies every four to five years to look for this condition. Though most people with chronic reflux never eventually develop cancer, the risk of cancer is higher for them than for the general population.

CORROSIVE INGESTION. Ingestion of a corrosive substance such as lye by children or adults (usually in suicide attempts) is extremely life threatening and requires the intervention of a gastroenterologist, surgeon and, typically, an intensive care unit. In some patients, corrosive ingestion leads immediately to death. However, if the corrosive agent is taken in a small amount or in a dilute form, patients may experience less penetrating injury and thus preserve their esophagus.

Some patients, because of the degree of injury at the onset from the toxin, form scars called strictures in the esophagus. These scars can lead to obstruction, reflux and an increased risk of esophageal cancer. All of these factors typically induce reflux in such patients.

CONGENITAL MALFORMATIONS. Congenital malformations are conditions present at birth. In some cases, congenital malformations that cause GERD are immediately obvious. More often, however, congenital malformations in the digestive tract do not cause problems until later in life.

Since digestion is an everyday occurrence, many people simply learn to live with digestive problems, assuming that the pain or difficulties they experience are normal. Later, a combination of other factors may lead them to seek medical attention. Then they discover that a part of the problem has been there all along.

Patients with congenital skeletal deformities of the bone, skin or internal organs may be at risk for disease. Some diseases may be associated with asymptomatic (no symptoms) reflux that can have long term significance, particularly in mentally disabled children or adults unable to give good medical histories or verbalize symptoms. In some conditions, endoscopy may be indicated in the appropriate clinical setting.

## Occupational Hazards

GERD can also be related to occupational hazards. In the aftermath of the September 11th, 2001 World Trade Center bombings in New York, 332 of the firefighters who survived soon developed what became known as the "World Trade Center Cough." According to a study by researcher David J. Prezant, reported in the September 12, 2002 issue of the New England Journal of Medicine, many firefighters had to take up to four weeks of sick leave following the disaster. Even among those who took very little sick leave for their cough, nearly all of these firefighters also developed acid reflux disease. The ones who had the worse problems were the ones who arrived at the scene first. In most cases, these firefighters did not have respirators and some did not even wear paper masks for the many hours they inhaled the thick smoke and debris that surrounded the crash site. Although this is a compelling report, and the first of which has ever been documented, it suggests that certain inhalants, such as those experienced and being studied at the World Trade Center site may also be causitive agents for acid reflux. Clearly, the jury is out on this, but it further suggests another of many atrocious effects of the terrorist attacks in New York City. It is unknown at this time if reflux disease will continue to be a problem for these firefighters in the years to come.

# 7

# THE ISSUE OF DIET
## *Identifying Problem Areas*

O NCE A DIAGNOSIS HAS BEEN MADE IDENTI-fying the probable causes of GERD, the doctor will talk to the patient about diet. Although there are many medications that are prescribed, most patients find that some subtle changes in diet can greatly impact and improve the painful symptoms of GERD. Diet rather than medication is by far the more important initial factor to consider in GERD management.

### Some Problem Foods

Perhaps no place on earth offers its citizens as much dietary diversity as does North America. Our citizens have the opportunity to choose from a huge variety of different foods and unlike many places in the world we can be assured that the foods we buy are clean and free from the diseases many people in third world countries regularly contract. Still, for those afflicted with GERD, even clean and abundant foods and beverages can make them sick. Likewise, no two people have quite the same reaction to the foods and beverages they put in their mouths. Some people can eat and drink just about anything and never seem to have a sick day in their lives. Other people suffer for days if they eat something just a little bit out of the ordinary.

Fortunately, for GERD sufferers, the list of problem foods is remarkably short.

CAFFEINATED BEVERAGES. All beverages that contain caffeine seem to cause problems for GERD sufferers. Caffeine has been shown to be a powerful stimulant in the production of stomach acid. Another problem with caffeine is its effect on the LES. Caffeine relaxes the sphincter, thereby allowing acid reflux to occur. Common caffeine-containing beverages include coffee, tea, hot chocolate, and soft drinks.

COFFEE. Fresh brewed coffee is very high in caffeine. An eight-ounce cup contains up to 120 milligrams. While decaffeinated coffee contains less caffeine, it is still a problem for GERD sufferers, since coffee is acidic and both irritates the stomach lining and stimulates the production of stomach acid. Switching to decaffeinated coffee is not enough to prevent reflux. It, unfortunately, can also cause significant reflux symptoms, even though it is less of a stimulant than caffeinated coffee.

TEA. Although tea has about half the caffeine of coffee, still it may contain enough to cause GERD symptoms. Currently there are also many herbal teas on the market. But just because a tea is labeled "herbal" doesn't mean that it's also caffeine free. Some are and some are not. Beware of "decaffeinated herbal teas," particularly those containing peppermint, mint, or other reflux-inducing ingredients.

HOT CHOCOLATE. Hot chocolate may be the ultimate comfort food on a cold, blustery night, but it's not a good beverage choice for a GERD sufferer. Chocolate tends to relax the LES and allows food from the stomach to reflux into the esophagus. Many people think that chocolate, in its pure form, contains caffeine. In truth, not all chocolate has caffeine and the chocolate that does contain caffeine usually contains negligible amounts. Theobromide, however, is a stimulant found in chocolate's pure form (cacao). This chemical, called a methyxanthine, acts as a stimulant and it can have caffeinelike effects, although these are less profound. Theobromide has not, however, been linked to gastroe-sophageal reflux disease.

SOFT DRINKS. Most colas (unless specifically labeled), as well as many other soft drinks, contain caffeine—even those sold in health food stores. Some soft drinks (including Jolt and Mountain Dew) contain very large quantities of caffeine. Before consuming a soft drink, be sure to read the label.

MINT. Mint has long been thought to aid the digestive process (hence the preponderance of after-dinner mints at restaurants). For people not subject to reflux, mint may be helpful since it encourages the burping up of the carbon dioxide formed in the digestive process. But for GERD sufferers that after-dinner mint or fragrant mint tea is generally more of a problem than a comfort since mint tends to reduce LES pressure and thus causes reflux. In some, mint (any type) is a potent stimulant of reflux.

VEGETABLES AND FRUITS. Most fruits and vegetables present no prob-lem for GERD sufferers. In fact, fruits and vegetables should form a major part of your diet. The only ones to should avoid are onions, toma-toes, and citrus juices. Those vegetables and fruits may be a problem because they can contain acetic acid or citric acid, which are potentially irritating to the lining of an esophagus that is already irritated by the acid refluxed from the stomach.

ALCOHOL. Alcohol presents several problems: It increases the flow of blood to the stomach, which in turn increases the production of stom-ach acid. Second, like tobacco smoke or very spicy foods, alcohol irri-tates the already inflamed tissues lining the esophagus and stomach. And third, alcohol is high in "empty" calories," calories with no food value. Alcohol also has a direct link to erosive esophagitis as well as to all can-cers of the upper GI tract.

## The Problem of Preparation

While many people have food allergies or intolerances to the foods mentioned above, for all people, the problem with food may not be so much the food itself, as it is the way it is prepared.

How does the preparation method affect the food? Take for example, one of America's most popular foods, the potato.

A whole, raw three-ounce potato contains about 65 calories and virtually no fat. Roasting that same potato in the oven with other foods, will probably add about 5 grams of fat and about 90 calories, for a total of 155 calories. Cut that same potato into large pieces and "home fry" them in a skillet with shortening or oil, and the result is a total of 12 grams of fat and 220 calories. Cut the potato into thinner strips or french fries and deep fry them in oil or shortening, and that three-ounce potato will end up with 15 grams of fat and 265 calories. Transform it into potato chips and that same three-ounce potato will end up with 30 grams of fat and 450 calories. (The Doctor's Pocket Calorie, Fat and Carbohydrate Counter, p6).

Fried foods are not only extremely high in calories and cholesterol, they also slow down gastric emptying and for many people that is sure to cause GERD. The longer food sits in the stomach, the more gastric acid is produced which then becomes available to reflux back into the esophagus. In addition when the stomach is full, it is often distended, which contributes to LES distention and poor closure of its valvelike opening. Poor closure of the LES also contributes to reflux.

When preparing a meal, GERD sufferers should choose methods of preparation that keep them healthy and also help them to avoid digestive upsets.

## Overeating

The average American eats too much food. To compound matters, most of that food is prepared in an unhealthful manner. The average portions served in American restaurants are prepared in such a way that they typically exceed our caloric needs for one meal.

These oversized portions are significantly larger than those in Europe, for example. According to a study published in the February 2002 edition of the American Journal of Public Health, a survey of New York restaurants revealed that a typical serving of pasta was three times the United States Department of Agriculture's recommended serving size.

The same is true for desserts. The portions are excessive, which contributes overall to the problem of obesity in the United States. And, of course, to reflux.

### Fast Food

Americans are notorious for eating high-fat junk food that is readily available at supermarkets and fast food outlets and promoted endlessly on television. The majority of the fast food available on a daily basis is loaded with fat, which greatly contributes to reflux in those who are prone to it.

A McDonald's Big Mac, for example has 590 calories and 34 grams of fat. An Arby's Italian Sub sandwich has 780 calories and 53 grams of fat. A six-ounce order of french fries has 540 calories and 25 grams of fat. A Taco Bell taco salad (if you eat the shell) has 850 calories and 52 grams of fat. A Nathan's Famous 4-piece chicken platter has 1790 calories and 109 grams of fat (The Doctor's Pocket Calorie, Fat & Carbohydrate Counter), and the list goes on.

As at other types of restaurants, serving sizes in fast food restaurants have been getting larger and larger. The basic McDonald's hamburger on a bun that started the fast-food revolution in the U.S. in the 1960s had about 340 calories and 16 grams of fat. The small (2.4 ounce) order of fries that came with it added about 210 calories, and the 12 oz. cola about 150 calories. Now it is not unusual for fast food restaurants to offer huge "super meals" like Burger King's Double Whopper meal. This sandwich has 1020 calories and 65 grams of fat, the side order of "super sized" fries contains more than 600 calories and nearly 30 grams of fat and the cola contains 150 calories per 12 ounces. Many "super-sized" soft drinks easily contain more than 36 oz. As you can see, in 40 years or so, our idea of a filling fast-food lunch has gone from 700 calories and 26 grams of fat to 1920 calories and 95 grams of fat. No wonder obesity is our fastest growing health problem!

THE ALL TOO TYPICAL AMERICAN DIET. The result of our tendency to make poor choices in both quantity of food as well as food preparation has led to what I consider to be a very poor typical daily American diet. It often looks something like this:

| MEAL | CALORIES | FAT | CARBS | FIBER | PROTEIN |
|---|---|---|---|---|---|
| **BREAKFAST** | | | | | |
| 2 slices of bacon | 80 | 7 | 0 | 0 | 4 |
| 2 fried eggs | 200 | 16 | 1 | 0 | 12 |
| 1 two-ounce Danish pastry | 220 | 10 | 25 | 0 | 0 |
| 2 cups of coffee | 0 | 0 | 0 | 0 | 0 |
| TOTAL | 500 | 33 | 26 | 0 | 16 |
| **LUNCH** | | | | | |
| Double Whopper | 590 | 34 | 47 | 2.5 | 150* |
| Large French fries | 540 | 25 | 72 | 6 | 5 |
| 1 22-ounce soft drink | 280 | 0 | 70 | 0 | 0 |
| TOTAL | 1410 | 59 | 156 | 8.50 | 115 |
| **BEFORE DINNER** | | | | | |
| 1 12-ounce can of beer | 140 | 0 | 3 | 0 | 1 |
| **DINNER** | | | | | |
| 2 pieces fried chicken | 400 | 24 | 8 | 0 | 50 |
| 1 cup mashed potatoes with gravy | 120 | 3 | 14 | 2 | 10 |

| | | | | | |
|---|---|---|---|---|---|
| 1 cup peas | 35 | 0 | 6 | 3 | 9 |
| 2 dinner rolls | 180 | 4 | 30 | 2 | 4 |
| 2 pats butter | 70 | 8 | 0 | 0 | 0 |
| 1 slice apple pie | 300 | 12 | 41 | 1 | 2 |
| 1 12-ounce soft drink | 150 | 0 | 37 | 0 | 0 |
| TOTAL | 1255 | 51 | 139 | 8.00 | 75 |
| **SNACK** | | | | | |
| 4 oz. of potato chips | 600 | 40 | 60 | 1 | 0 |
| 1 22-ounce soft drink | 280 | 0 | 37 | 0 | 0 |
| TOTAL FOR DAY | 4187 | 183 | 418 | 17.5 | 207 |
| CALORIES FROM FAT, CARBOHYDRATE OR PROTEIN | | 1647 | 1672 | | 868 |
| PERCENTAGES OF CALORIES FROM FAT, CARBOHYDRATES OR PROTEINS | | 40% | 39% | | 20% |

In Chapter 8 we'll take a look at what a healthier diet might look like.

It is generally agreed that we could easily sustain good health by consuming between 1,500 and 2,400 calories a day (depending on age, gender, activity level, muscle mass, and other factors); however, many of us (as illustrated by the diet above) take in many more. And, in doing so, eat a diet that contains more than 30 percent more protein and 20 percent more fat than necessary, very little fruit, not enough fiber, and a poor balance between fats and carbohydrates. Being overweight and eating too much at a time are two major contributing factors to GERD.

## Sedentary Lifestyle

Most Americans live comparatively sedentary lives. We drive or ride rather than walk to work or to school and we spend too much time on the couch watching television. If you suffer from GERD you need to be careful about what type of exercise you do. If your current diet resembles the one described above, you are in serious need of additional exercise. A pound of fat in your body is worth about 3,500 calories. To lose one pound a week, you will need to eliminate at least

500 calories a day. You won't do that lying on the sofa or sitting in front of your computer.

## Processed Foods

Processed foods can also be a problem for those suffering from GERD. Preservatives and other additives have revolutionized our economy by making our food distribution system possible and allowing us to get just about any food any time of year. But we have paid a price. The chemicals added to much of our food may be difficult for many of us to digest. As a result, our food tends to remain in our digestive tracts for a longer period of time. This means a longer period of bacterial digestion, which produces gas. The gas expands, forcing the LES open, subsequently causing gas and acid to reflux into esophagus.

When this happens, it would seem logical to take an antacid, but, in fact, that may only exacerbate the problem. The antacid will make the stomach stop producing acid just when it needs more acid to digest the food that remains. This starts a vicious cycle in which the stomach will then produce even more acid in order to compensate for that requirement.

The most common food additives are monosodium glutamate (MSG), aspartame, and saccharin. Other additives include antioxidants, binders, catalysts, colorings, flavor enhancers, flavorings, gelifiers, lubricants, preservatives, propulsive agents, solvents, stabilizers, sweeteners, thickeners, unmolding agents, and yeast. These additives have very little nutritional value and are potentially harmful in large quantities. Their purpose is to add flavor and for preservative effect. Our advice is to try as much as possible to eat natural (preferably organic) foods, because there is increased likelihood that you will eat food with maximal nutrients and minimal artificial additives. This will likely make you feel better and make you healthier in the long run.

## Food Intolerance

GERD tends to be a chronic disease and some foods—particularly milk products and wheat—seem to consistently cause chemical reactions in the body that result in GERD and other intestinal problems. There are now several products on the market, such as Lactaid and soy, that can help a patient overcome these intolerances. However, we generally recommend that patients consider simply eliminating those foods from their diets, if possible. Fortunately, there is an increasing number of soy products that can be substituted for milk products. Corn, rice, spelt and other grains can be substituted for wheat. (The Web site www.ener-g.com may be a useful resource for those looking for wheat-free products.)

## Food Allergies

In some patients, the problem is not a food intolerance but a food allergy, although the symptoms are similar. In the case of intolerance, the problem is created by an adverse chemical reaction. In the case of an allergy, the immune system becomes involved, sensing the food as a foreign substance that must be destroyed or removed from the body. Because true food allergies can result in dangerous reactions, including diarrhea, intestinal cramping, swelling, and vomiting, it is important that the specific cause of the reaction be diagnosed and the problem foods be eliminated from the diet. Although allergies and intolerances are not directly related to GERD, there can be considerable overlap and these intolerances can often be difficult to characterize. Pay attention to the foods you eat and how you respond to them. Often times patients have a better sense of their intolerances than their physicians. Such patients usually have already eliminated such foods from their diets prior to even visiting their physician. Others, however, will discover the source of their problem only by keeping an accurate food diary.

## Fad Diets

Thanks again to the abundance and variety of delicious foods we enjoy, many Americans are significantly overweight. To correct this problem many turn to fad diets. While we certainly recommend that everyone try to achieve a healthy weight, we never recommend fad diets. Rather, it is the physician's job to help patients change life-long poor eating habits and recognize the importance of exercise.

Fad diets seldom work for more than a short period of time and most can trigger episodes of GERD.

HIGH-FAT, LOW-CARBOHYDRATE DIETS. The theory behind these diets is that significantly reducing carbohydrates and increasing protein intake speeds metabolism and allows you to lose weight quickly. This is based on a theory that ketosis is a form of fat burning that occurs in the absence of carbohydrates. While many people may indeed effectively lose weight on this diet, drastically changing one's diet in this manner can be difficult for many. These diets are very unbalanced and are extremely high in fat with side effects often including nausea, fatigue, fluid loss and the potential for kidney problems. Like all fad diets, once you return to a normal eating pattern, the likelihood is that you will regain all the weight you have lost, and perhaps even more.

HIGH-CARBOHYDRATE DIETS. These diets are based on the theory that eating carbohydrates during a specific time of the day will decrease the production of insulin, which leads to fewer calories giving way to fat cells. It was originally thought that by decreasing fat intake and replacing it with carbohydrates, one could burn the carbohydrates since they were the easiest substances to break down and convert to sugars for fuel. The problem with the theory is that most people who consume high-carbohydrate diets end up eating too many calories. Those excess calories, if not utilized as energy, get stored as fat. Because this diet is unbalanced, short-term loss will usually result in long-term gain.

FASTING. Fasting is another way many people choose to lose weight quickly. While short-term fasting to "detoxify" the body for religious or spiritual reasons may be relatively harmless, fasting on a long-term basis can rob the body of essential vitamins and minerals and cause food cravings. This is an unrealistic form of weight control and almost always results in return to eating the same if not more than what was previously eaten.

SINGLE FOOD DIETS. Over the years, many fad diets have also depended on eating one food or type of food at every meal. One of the most well publicized of these diets was the "Mayo Clinic Diet" (which, in fact, was never endorsed by the famous clinic). This diet was comprised of eating grapefruit with every meal. A certain amount of fruit everyday is a good idea, but a single-food approach is a difficult one to maintain for extended periods of time.

OTHER DIETS. For a variety of reasons, some relating to health, some to environmental concerns, some religious beliefs, some cultural, many Americans now adhere to diets that require abstinence from some of the foods recommended by the USDA's food pyramid. These include:

MACROBIOTIC DIETS. Macrobiotic diets first became widespread in the 1960s as part of the trend toward more "natural" foods and eating according to the environment in which you live. Those who follow this diet try to eliminate all processed foods, substituting whole grains, greens, beans, seeds, roots and fruit. While a macrobiotic diet can be healthy, it is quite regimented and in most cases limits its followers to foods prepared at home. In general, macrobiotic diets are healthy and can result in adequate intake of essential vitamins and minerals. However, it requires a great deal of dedication and is difficult to maintain for the average American.

VEGETARIAN AND/OR VEGAN DIETS. If you were an alien from outer space getting all your information about the American diet from television commercials, you would surely conclude that we subsist primarily on hamburgers. While the majority of Americans probably do eat at a variety of meat and meat products, many people live very healthy lives eating no red meat (but chicken and fish), or no meat at all. Because of the widespread availability of vegetables, grains, nuts and seeds, even a strict vegetarian diet can be very healthy.

Vegans differ from vegetarians in that they eliminate not only meat from their diet, but also all dairy products, eggs, fish, honey, and all other animal products or animal derivatives. While it would do all of us a lot of good to restrict the amount of meat in our diets, if you do so, or eliminate meat altogether, it is important to supplement with other foods that provide the proteins you need to balance your diet.

There is no evidence that any of these diets actually make GERD symptoms worse or induce the symptoms of GERD. The primary culprits I mentioned earlier have been shown to worsen GERD regardless of whether or not they are taken in patients who eat strict macrobiotic, vegetarian or vegan diets.

## Timing

In addition to what we eat, when and how we eat can also have an effect on GERD. For too many of us, a typical day includes grabbing a pastry and a cup of coffee on the way out the door, fast food at our desks for lunch, a couple of snacks during the day, a heavy dinner in the evening, and more snacks right before bed. Each of these practices is a recipe for GERD. One important step GERD patients can take is to avoid high-fat foods on the run, in large quantities, or late in the evening.

# 8

# HEALTHY EATING
# & GERD
## *Making Better Choices*

S INCE ELIMINATING GERD FROM YOUR LIFE
may involve changing the way you now eat, there are some
things you might want to know about nutrition in general
and the role good nutrition plays in controlling GERD.

### *What is Good Nutrition?*

Since eating is such an important part of life, it is probably little wonder that over the centuries there have been many theories about what
constitutes the perfect diet. For people in many parts of the world, the
answer is simple: Nutrition—good or bad—consists of whatever they
can get. In fact, a large percentage of the world's population still exists
primarily on rice, beans, lentils, a few vegetables, and an occasional
fish or chicken.

For us the answer is more complex. Unlike the millions of under-
nourished people in the world, most of us have ready access to just
about anything we want. Our dietary dilemma is different—not how

to get enough to eat, but how to make healthy choices from among the many foods that are available.

Since the early 1900s, as a society we have already made several major changes in what we eat. According to the United States Department of Agriculture (USDA), between 1910 and 1976, wheat consumption in the U.S. dropped by 48 percent, corn by 85 percent, rye by 78 percent, barley by 66 percent, buckwheat by 98 percent, and beans and legumes by 46 percent. There has also been a 23 percent decrease in the consumption of fresh vegetables and a 33 percent decrease in the consumption of fresh fruit.

The modernization of food production, particularly with the introduction of canned, frozen, and packaged foods, along with the assembly line production of all supermarket food, has resulted in decreased consumption of many of the older grain foods and fruits that once were common staples of the American diet.

Grains, once considered among the basic sources of nutrition, have now been replaced by foods such as meat, chicken, and cheese. In the U.S. and wherever methods of food production and agriculture are modernized, much of our grain products are now used to feed cattle, not people. Within the 60 years of decreased grain production the actual consumption of beef has risen by 72 percent, poultry by 194 percent, and cheese by 322 percent.

Further, as we have moved away from farms and small towns, preparing fresh food can now actually be more expensive and less convenient for many people in industrialized societies. Thus within the last 60 years, consumption of canned vegetables has increased by 320 percent, frozen vegetables by 1,650 percent, and processed fruit by 556 percent in the U.S. alone. Along with canning and freezing foods is the addition of chemical additives to the food supply, which has increased by a staggering figure of 995 percent since 1940. Our consumption of beverages has also markedly changed. Water and milk consumption has declined from 60 years ago, while soft drink consumption has increased by 2,638 percent.

## *What Should We Eat?*

There has been a great deal of debate regarding what should constitute a healthy American diet. There is now criticism about the lack of useful information in the USDA's traditional Food Guide Pyramid that appears in textbooks and on the packaging of food products. Of particular concern is its lack of a stance on higher protein foods, lower carbohydrate products, and lower fat intake recommendations, as well as its lack of information about the types of bread, fruits, meat, or grains, that should be part of a healthy diet.

Although the food pyramid has not been updated since 1996 and does not discuss questions that now arise in more current food health issues, it still remains an important guideline since it continues to stress the need for a balance between carbohydrates, protein and fat intake. But people today are more interested than ever in not only

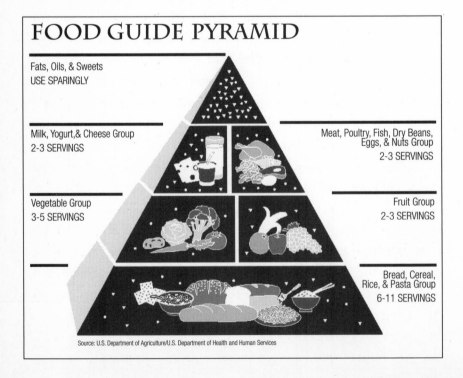

# FOOD GUIDE PYRAMID

Fats, Oils, & Sweets
USE SPARINGLY

Milk, Yogurt,& Cheese Group
2-3 SERVINGS

Meat, Poultry, Fish, Dry Beans, Eggs, & Nuts Group
2-3 SERVINGS

Vegetable Group
3-5 SERVINGS

Fruit Group
2-3 SERVINGS

Bread, Cereal, Rice, & Pasta Group
6-11 SERVINGS

Source: U.S. Department of Agriculture/U.S. Department of Health and Human Services

knowing about the groups of foods they should eat but specifically what types of grains, meat, or fruits are best, since current evidence suggests that there are important differences among many of the choices in each "family" of foods.

In September 2002, The Institute of Medicine of the National Academy of Science published a 1,000-page report issuing for the first time recommendations about "micronutrients" (proteins, fats, and carbohydrates) along with suggestions about how much dietary fiber people should consume. Before reviewing this newer report, let us recall the USDA's earlier recommendations.

The traditional Food Guide Pyramid is divided into six food groups, five of which include foods the USDA recommends we should have at least some of every day to meet generally accepted guidelines for good health. The sixth group, fats and sweets, is the group we should indulge in only once in awhile.

## What Constitutes a Serving?

The first thing you'll notice in studying the Food Guide Pyramid is that its recommendations in each category of foods is given not in weight or volume, but in "servings." At first glance, one might think that meeting the USDA's standards would mean eating a great deal of food. The typical American "serving" size, however, has gotten progressively larger, so that our modern day concept of a "serving" is probably very different from that of the USDA's recommendation. For instance, in a typical American restaurant, one serving of pasta is three cups. According to the Food Guide Pyramid, one serving of pasta should be 1/2 cup—quite a difference.

According to the Food Guide Pyramid, one serving equals:

| BREAD, CEREAL, RICE, PASTA | MILK/MILK ALTERNATIVES |
|---|---|
| 1 slice bread<br>1/2 bun or English muffin<br>4 small crackers or 1 tortilla<br>1 ounce ready-to-eat cereal<br>1/2 cup cooked cereal, rice, or pasta | 1 cup milk, soy drink, or yogurt<br>1 1/2 ounces cheese<br>1/2 cup cottage cheese |
| FRUIT | MEAT/MEAT ALTERNATIVES |
| 1 medium apple, orange or banana<br>1/2 cup canned fruit<br>1/4 cup dried fruit<br>3/4 cup fruit juice<br>1/4 medium avocado | 2–3 ounces cooked lean<br>    meat/poultry/fish<br>2 eggs, 7 ounces tofu, or 1/2 cup nuts<br>1 cup cooked dried beans or chickpeas |
| VEGETABLE | FATS, SWEETS AND OILS |
| 1 cup raw leafy vegetables<br>1/2 cup raw chopped vegetables<br>1/2 cup cooked vegetables<br>1/2 to 3/4 cup vegetable juice | Only occasional small servings |

These recommendations are excellent reminders of the need to decrease food portions. This older emphasis on portion size is an important one particularly in an age where excess in just about every activity has become commonplace in American society. In fact, at an early age most children should be taught much more about nutrition so that by the time they are young adults they will understand that balancing these foods in both substance and quantity will benefit them in other activities throughout their lives.

The food pyramid plan is, however, still not specific enough for the American food consumer. Whether they live on a farm in Iowa or the middle of bustling New York City, people are now more concerned than ever about what types of foods are best for their health. They now want to know specifically what the caloric values in different versions of the same food are, in foods such as milk products, whey, and animal proteins, and, certainly, the amount of fat.

Some diet plans, such as the Atkins diet, advocate that protein foods replace carbohydrates for caloric energy. These unbalanced diets can result in quick weight loss, but for most people they ultimately result in recurrent weight gain when a more balanced diet is resumed.

For the majority of Americans, the only proven way to lose weight permanently is by adhering to a healthy, balanced diet with an emphasis on minimizing consumption of excessive calories. A normal amount of exercise, which can be little more that a regular walking program, may also go a long way in helping weight management as well as improving the digestive process.

Many Americans wonder, "I'm eating a well balanced diet low in total fat percentages, so why can't I lose weight?" What they don't realize is that continuous overconsumption of even so-called healthy foods will result in a weight gain and increased body fat composition. Two large bowls of pasta a day, for example, can significantly add to daily caloric intake if eaten in addition to other normal or high-calorie meals. Remember, the recommended single serving of pasta is 1/2 cup, six times less than what the average American consumes at a restaurant.

## A Calorie is a Calorie is a Calorie

A calorie is a calorie no matter what its source. If you're trying to keep your weight constant, you need to burn the same number of calories you take in. If you are trying to lose weight, you need to burn more calories than you are taking in.

Because calories are so important to a discussion of a balanced diet, however, it is important to remember what a calorie is. The scientific definition of a calorie is the amount of heat needed to raise the temperature of one liter of water one degree centigrade. Calories are the way we measure the energy-producing value in food as it is oxidized in the body to produce energy. Therefore, when we compare fat calories to carbohydrates or protein, for example, it's important to recognize how much energy each of these three food types require to burn let's say a gram of each type of food. That is, how many calories does it take to break down that gram of food?

Certainly you could fuel your body with calories from just one source. For example, you could consume 2,000 calories by eating ten 200-calorie chocolate bars. While this might be enjoyable at first, the all-candy bar diet would be unbalanced (and would almost certainly result in GERD!) and unlikely to satisfy your food cravings and hunger in a 24-hour period. It is true that if you did eat 10 chocolate bars in a day (not unheard of for some Americans) you would have fulfilled all the required daily caloric needs for your body to function. The problem is, those 10 chocolate bars would have offered few if any of the essential vitamins and minerals required to maintain a healthy and functioning body, and they certainly would not have helped you take in the number of carbohydrates and proteins you need.

Instead, nutritionists have determined that to maintain good health, you should try to balance your diet each day with particular percentages of calories from the various food groups in the food pyramid. According to this formula, you're allowed more servings of some foods than others because some foods have more calories than others. For example, a gram of protein or carbohydrate contains only four calories, while a gram of fat contains nine. So the higher the fat content of a food, the more calories (or amount of energy it will take) to break one gram of it down. A general guideline is that fats contain about 120 calories per tablespoonful.

To balance your diet—that is, achieve what nutritionists consider the healthiest combination of fats, proteins, and carbohydrates—you need to consider the proportion of each that occurs in food.

In all foods you eat, you get more than double the calories from fat than you do from protein and carbohydrates. To determine exactly how many calories you are getting from the fat, protein, and carbohydrates in various foods, you multiply the number of grams of fat by nine and the number of grams of carbohydrates and protein by four.

For example, one cup of whole milk contains 148 calories, derived from 8 grams of fat, 8 grams of protein and 11 grams of carbohydrate. If you multiply the 8 grams of fat by 9, you discover that 72 of the calories in the milk came from fat. If you multiply the 8 grams of protein by 4, you find that 32 of the calories in the milk came from protein. And if you multiply the 11 grams of carbohydrate by 4, you find that 44 of the calories in milk came from carbohydrate.

Most nutritionists suggest that you consume 20 to 30 percent of your daily caloric intake from fat, 15 to 20 percent from protein, and 50 to 65 percent from carbohydrates. Since most adults require 2,000 to 3,000 calories a day, that would mean that your daily caloric intake should be balanced as follows:

| CALORIES PER DAY | 2,000 3,000 |
| --- | --- |
| PROTEIN CALORIES | 300 to 400 450 to 600 |
| FAT CALORIES | 400 to 600 600 to 900 |
| CARBOHYDRATE CALORIES | 1000 to 1300 1500 to 1950 |

## Nutrition Facts

Serving Size 1/2 cup dry (40g)
Servings Per Container 30

**Amount Per Serving**

**Calories** 150    Calories from Fat 25

| | % Daily Value* |
| --- | --- |
| **Total Fat** 3g | 5% |
| Saturated Fat 0.5g | 2% |
| Polyunsaturated Fat 1g | |
| Monounsaturated Fat 1g | |
| **Cholesterol** 0mg | 0% |
| **Sodium** 0mg | 0% |
| **Total Carbohydrate** 27g | 9% |
| Dietary Fiber 4g | 15% |
| Sugars 1g | |
| **Protein** 5g | |

| | |
| --- | --- |
| Vitamin A | 0% |
| Vitamin C | 0% |
| Calcium | 0% |
| Iron | 10% |

* Percent Daily Values are based on a 2,000 calorie diet. Your Daily Values may be higher or lower depending on your calorie needs:

| | Calories: | 2,000 | 2,500 |
| --- | --- | --- | --- |
| Total Fat | Less than | 65g | 80g |
| Sat Fat | Less than | 20g | 25g |
| Cholesterol | Less than | 300mg | 300mg |
| Sodium | Less than | 2,400mg | 2,400mg |
| Total Carbohydrate | | 300g | 375g |
| Dietary Fiber | | 25g | 30g |

According to a September, 2002, National Academy of Science study, a "healthy" diet is comprised of 20 to 35 percent fat, 10 to 35 percent protein and 45 to 60 percent carbohydrates. These recommendations differ slightly from those above, suggesting slightly more protein and a little less carbohydrate. The recommendation about fat is about the same. The report also recommends that "added" sugars comprise no more than 25 percent of total calories.

Few foods, of course are purely protein, fat, or carbohydrate. For example, a baked potato contains 5 grams of protein, 51 grams of carbohydrate and no fat. Three ounces (one FDA serving) of roasted ham contains 21 grams of protein, 5 grams of fat, and no carbohydrates. A cup of plain macaroni contains 5 grams of protein, 1 gram of fat, and 32 grams of carbohydrates. That means it's important to eat a variety of foods.

Also, it is important to remember that to eat a healthy diet, you must consider the diet as a whole rather than any one component of it. For example, many people avoid some foods—avocados, nuts, seeds—that are high in fat but that are actually quite beneficial to health. Peanut butter, for example, is a high-fat product. But a lunch consisting of a peanut butter and jelly sandwich on whole wheat bread, an apple, and a carton of low-fat yogurt has an overall fat content that is fairly low. The fat taken in would actually be much healthier than the same amount of fat that is in a bag of potato chips, for example. Plus, you would avoid the artificial preservatives in the chips that add no nutritional value.

As you are getting used to eating a healthy, balanced diet, we suggest you identify a good diet source or cookbook that uses a table of foods listing the percentages of carbohydrates, proteins and fat found in each type of food and do the calculations to discover the percentages of protein, carbohydrates and fats in your diet. Cookbooks such as The Joy of Cooking do contain such charts.

## Food Labels

It is wise to be conscientious about reading the labels that, by law, must now appear on most packaged foods and beverages. For example, if you look at this label for Quaker® Oats, you will see that it includes the serving size, the number of calories in one serving, and information about the percentages of fat, cholesterol, sodium, carbohydrates, proteins, and vitamins the product contains, along with the percentages of the USDA recommended amounts one serving would contain.

It is particularly important to read the labels on processed foods and over-the-counter medicines because many contain products such as tomatoes, acids and caffeine that are of particular concern to those who suffer from GERD.

## *More about Fat*

Fat is important to a balanced diet since it supplies much of the energy you need to maintain an active lifestyle and is a very important fuel used by the body to maintain its integral functions. Rather than trying to limit your fat completely, as many dieters think they should do, instead I would advise you to concentrate on limiting yourself to the "healthy" fats described below.

Not surprisingly, the amount of fat desirable varies from individual to individual and for the same individuals of different ages. The chart below is a helpful guide to the generally accepted amount of fat suggested per day. Please note that this is a recommended gram percentage not to be exceeded.

Many physicians and nutritionists today may suggest even lower quantities of fat intake. There is some controversy among dieticians regarding this point, but we do know that the following limitations do significantly reduce long-term effects of fat intake.

Healthy ranges for fat intake are as follows.

| | |
|---|---|
| CHILDREN | 30 TO 60G |
| TEENAGERS | 0 TO 80G |
| WOMEN | 30 TO 60G |
| MEN | 40 TO 80G |
| ATHLETES | 80 TO 120G |

TYPES OF FATS. Because fat intake is such an important component of a healthy diet, it is very important that we understand that not all fats are equally good for us. What are the differences in the fats we consume?

There are four primary types of fats in the foods we eat: saturated fats, monounsaturated fats, polyunsaturated fats, and trans fats (sometimes referred to as trans fatty acids). In general, saturated fats remain solid at room temperature (exceptions are palm and coconut oils). Saturated fats include foods such as lard, butter, suet, margarine, and the fat that is "marbled" in meat.

Monounsaturated and polyunsaturated fats are generally liquid at room temperature, but will solidify if you refrigerate them. These unsaturated fats are found in foods including canola, corn, and olive oil; nuts, seeds, avocado, and soy. They are also found in fish such as salmon, tuna, mackerel, trout, and sardines.

Trans fats are both synthetically manufactured and occur naturally in some foods. When they are synthetically produced, they are made by adding hydrogen to fats, usually to solidify them to give them a longer shelf life. Products that are described as "hydrogenated" contain trans fats. Many processed and packaged foods contain a high percentage of these trans fatty acids.

There is still some controversy about exactly what effect fats have on the body (and new and sometime conflicting studies appear regularly). But in general, it is a good idea to try to avoid as many saturated and trans fats as possible since they raise the level of cholesterol and increase the risk of certain cancers. I would consider these "bad fats" whereas the other fats mentioned are "good fats." Although at the time this book was written there was a growing controversy about the role of trans fats in heart disease, certainly a high fat diet including too much of any kind of fat does seem to contribute to obesity—a major problem for people with GERD.

To maintain a healthy diet, including achieving a healthy weight, it is important to balance your food intake among fats, carbohydrates and proteins. Since most trans fats are found in processed foods it is often difficult to figure out just what percentage of any prepared food is composed of fat. Your best options are, whenever possible, to prepare your meals from fresh ingredients, use low-fat alternatives such as cooking sprays (instead of shortening), steam or broil foods instead of frying them and stay away from as much junk food as possible.

## *More about Carbohydrates*

Carbohydrates are the components of our foods that contain starch and fiber. When we ingest carbohydrates, our bodies break the starch down into the glucose that provides us with energy. Carbohydrates are basically chains of many sugars all linked together. However, it is important to note in this discussion of carbohydrates, that although they are comprised of many simple sugars linked together, they should not be confused with refined sugar, which will be discussed in the next section.

Like fats, carbohydrates are also divided into categories. Simple carbohydrates (monosaccharides) are found naturally in foods such as fruit and honey. Complex carbohydrates are found naturally in vegetables, rice, grains and beans.

SUGAR. The National Academy of Sciences (NAS) report mentioned earlier also concluded that up to 25% of daily calories in a healthy diet could be derived from sugars such as those added to processed foods, soft drinks and ice cream. While it may be true that in our junk-food society many people DO ingest at least that much sugar, this aspect of the NAS study is sure to cause considerable controversy, particularly since so many Americans are already obese. Other organizations such as the Center for Science in the Public Interest, recommend that less than a 10% daily intake of calories from sugar is a more desirable number. However this debate is eventually settled, there is little doubt that refined sugar is a source of calories that can easily be decreased in patients who wish to lose weight. Even in those patients who do not need to lose weight, keeping sugar consumption low will lead to a much more balanced and healthier diet.

## More about Protein

Protein is important because it builds and repairs muscles. Proteins are also the most important chemical stimulants of acid secretion in the stomach. Yet protein also acts as a buffer, since it is amphoteric— that is, stimulates acids and yet neutralizes acids at the same time. So protein's "good" and "bad" qualities balance each other out.

Although muscles are made largely of protein, protein is not what muscles use for fuel. They use carbohydrates and fats. Therefore, contrary to many dietary theories, adding a lot of excess protein to the diet does not increase strength or endurance. Whatever proteins the body can't use are eliminated by the body.

Weight lifters are an exception to this rule, however, as they tend to hold onto more of the protein they take in as they require more protein as a building block of muscle growth and development. Weight lifters, particularly heavy weight lifters, cause trauma and injury to the muscle and destroy muscle fibers intentionally to "rebuild" the muscle. The excessive strain of the muscle fibers with heavy lifting allows for growth and development of the muscles affected. In order for these metabolic processes to occur, extra energy intake is required in the form of calories to increase muscle strength and size. The building blocks of proteins (amino acids) are also required for muscles to form and develop and to allow for further muscle development.

If you're not a weight lifter (and perhaps even if you are), however, it is important to note that excess protein intake can be dangerous because it can damage organs such as the kidneys in patients with other predisposing conditions affecting these organs.

FIBER. Although, unlike many other mammals, we cannot digest fiber, it is nonetheless very important to digestion. Fiber absorbs water and helps move other indigestible substances through the colon. Fiber is an important substance that helps to bulk the stool and often allows for formed bowel movements. Intake of fiber can reduce the likelihood of constipation and is often recommended in patients with straining and difficult passage of stool. Although a balanced diet does contain fiber, in people over the age of 50, an additional fiber supplement may be recommended.

VITAMINS. Look at any food label, such as the one on page 71, you will notice that in addition to information about fats, proteins, and carbohydrates, it also includes the percentage of "recommended daily allowances" for vitamins found in the product.

This recommended daily allowance (RDA) was created by the National Academy of Sciences in 1941 for the War Department as the standard for the meals prepared for soldiers and has remained the standard ever since. Since this standard was created for teenaged boys, we can assume that it would represent the maximum amount of vitamins anyone would need. So, if you're not a teenaged boy, or you have a particular disease or medical condition, your doctor may recommend a slightly different dosage. Since World War II, the federal government has updated its recommendations about appropriate vitamin intake; those recommendations are called the Recommended Daily Intake (RDI).

Vitamins are chemicals found in food that regulate metabolic processes in the body. Dozens of specific vitamins have been identified and are classified alphabetically (e.g., vitamin A, vitamin, B, etc.). Vitamins in the human body are further categorized by the substance in which they are broken down. Thus, vitamins are either fat-soluble or water-soluble. The fat-soluble vitamins (A, D, E and K) can be stored in the body, but the water-soluble vitamins (B and C) cannot be stored and must be continuously replenished.

If you eat a healthy diet including a variety of the foods recommended by the Food Guide Pyramid, chances are you will not require additional vitamin supplements. In fact, if over-consumed, some vitamins can build to harmful levels in your body.

Excess amounts of vitamins will also be eliminated by the human body, particularly if the excess amounts are taken by mouth. Many people who already have well balanced diets do not need vitamin supplements. Interestingly, in our culture, many people nonetheless take excess expensive and unnecessary vitamins because they feel that it may help them, when oftentimes they do no good and potentially can do harm. If you are taking vitamins, or if you are considering adding vitamin supplements to your diet, ask your doctor for a recommendation about what vitamins are right for you or if they are necessary at all.

Some healthy people with well-balanced diets do need vitamin supplementation, however. These are usually people with diseases that affect their bodies and require vitamins to prevent problems. An example of such a disease is primary biliary cirrhosis, an unusual condition of the liver that can be associated with vitamin deficiencies and osteoporosis. In these patients vitamin supplements are given even when they eat a well-balanced diet.

MINERALS. Minerals, like vitamins, are essential for good health. Minerals help the muscles contract, the cells breathe, and maintain the balance in the body between acids and bases. Minerals we need include calcium, chloride, chromium, copper, fluoride, iodine, iron, magnesium, magnesium, molybdenum, phosphorus, potassium, selenium, sodium, and zinc. Again, eating a balanced diet should provide you with all the minerals your body needs, but if you are pregnant or have specific diseases or medical conditions, your doctor may recommend that you take additional minerals. Too many of some minerals can be harmful, so it is important to ask your doctor before you add more of them to your diet.

## Weight Control

Being overweight by more than 20 percent is not healthy for anyone, but it is particularly undesirable for people with GERD. Earlier in this chapter, we discussed the recommendations of the Food Guide Pyramid, including the types of food and serving sizes. Those recommendations are for people who are of the correct weight for their height and age. What is the correct weight for your height and age?

Achieving the "right" weight is a matter of great controversy. Although we doctors advise our patients to avoid becoming obese, we are also very concerned when our patients try to achieve the underweight proportions of the models on magazine covers. Similarly, we become concerned when our older patients try to maintain the same weight to height ratio as teenaged boys and girls. Thus, we suggest that you try to keep your weight somewhere near that suggested on the following chart.

USDA SUGGESTED WEIGHTS (HARVARD GUIDE TO WOMEN'S HEALTH, 648)
  Women and Men

| HEIGHT WITHOUT SHOES | WEIGHT W/O CLOTHES [19-34 years old] | WEIGHT W/O CLOTHES [Over 35 years old] |
|---|---|---|
| 5'0" | 97–128 | 111–137 |
| 5'1" | 101–132 | 111–143 |
| 5'2" | 104–137 | 115–148 |
| 5'3" | 107–141 | 119–152 |
| 5'4" | 111–146 | 122–157 |
| 5'5" | 114–150 | 126–162 |
| 5'6" | 118–155 | 130–167 |
| 5'7" | 121–160 | 134–170 |
| 5'8" | 125–164 | 138–178 |
| 5'9" | 129–169 | 142–183 |
| 5'10" | 132–174 | 146–188 |
| 5'11" | 136–179 | 151–194 |
| 6'0" | 140–184 | 155–199 |

As you can see by this chart, some weight gain can be anticipated after age 35. Also, since the bones and muscles of men tend to weigh more than women, the healthy weight for a woman would be at the lower end of the scale and the healthy weight for a man is toward the upper end of the scale.

If you would benefit from losing weight, you may need to modify your diet in several ways, because, despite what the many purveyors of miracle weight loss plans claim, the only way to lose weight is to consume fewer calories or burn more calories than you take in. A pound of fat in food or in our bodies is worth about 3,500 calories. To lose one pound each week requires a daily consuming 500 calories less than you do now and/or exercising more. Happily, as you will discover Chapter 9, a brisk four-mile walk can burn those 500 calories.

Of course, losing weight is not that simple, particularly since we Americans often eat out and even at home eat many prepackaged foods. When making decisions about what to include in your diet, for a while, at least, you'll want to refer often to a chart that lists the protein, carbohydrate and fat composition of various foods and ingredients, since some foods can really surprise you. For example, while most fruits are low in fat and calories, 1/2 cup of avocado contains 185 calories and 18 grams of fat. A cup of coconut contains 283 calories and a whopping 27 grams of fat—only 10 calories and 9 grams of fat more than a 3-ounce hamburger.

If you have a significant amount of weight to lose, your best strategy would be to consult with your doctor or a registered dietician. Together, they can help you plan a healthy and balanced diet combined with a sensible exercise regimen that will allow you to take off the pounds you need to and keep them off.

## 12 Rules for Living with GERD

For many years it was though that the only way to avoid the symptoms of GERD was to consume only bland foods. While there are still several foods that should be avoided, there is no reason why a diet that is good for your stomach and esophagus can't be healthy and enjoyable, as well.

So, what can you eat? Just about anything you want, with perhaps a few exceptions that vary from one person to another. But you should follow the rules listed below:

RULE 1: *Don't deep fry anything.* Fried foods are loaded with calories, and fats are the hardest things for your stomach to digest. Does that mean you are doomed forever to a life without french fries? No. It just means that, like other high-calorie, high-fat foods, you should consider placing them at the top of your food pyramid with the other foods you eat sparingly.

RULE 2: *Measure and count.* Because being overweight contributes to GERD, you may need to lose a few pounds. To do this, you need to restrict the number of calories you take in to less than the number of calories you burn each day. To figure out how many calories you take in, you need to count the calories in everything you eat and add them up at the end of each day. As we mentioned in previous chapters, appropriate calorie intake depends on age, gender, activity level, muscle mass, overall health, and other factors, as well. So, before starting any weight loss program, consult your doctor and/or a registered dietician.

RULE 3: *Keep a food diary.* Take a food diary on your first visit to your doctor, then continue to keep the diary. In it, record everything you put in your mouth from the time you get up until you go to bed (including gum and water). Buy yourself a cookbook or guidebook (they are available at all bookstores) that lists the percentages of fats, carbohydrates, and protein in foods and at the end of each day, add up your daily intake. Just about all foods have a label that lists total serving calories, ingredients, percentages of fat, cholesterol, carbohydrates, protein, and sugar as well as vitamins and minerals. Make it a habit to read those labels on every item you purchase. You will be amazed by how many calories some products advertised as "low calorie" or "low fat" actually contain. Try to be diligent about keeping your food diary for at least a month. Most people eat a lot more snacks, junk, and fatty foods than they think. It may surprise you to see how much you are actually eating each day.

The diary is an important first step in eating more healthily. After you've kept the food diary for a month you will be able to see what your eating patterns really are. You can then begin to make the adjustments you need to achieve fewer symptoms of GERD and lose weight.

RULE 4: *Set goals.* There isn't much reason to keep a diary if you haven't set some goals for yourself. Ask your doctor or a registered dietician to help you decide what you could realistically expect to change about your current dietary habits that would help you avoid the foods and dietary habits that have led to your GERD. For example, take one item that you know is a "weakness," focus on it, overcome it, and move on to the next. It may take months (or even years), but you are more likely to achieve the results you want if you gradually transition out of bad habits one at a time until you achieve your ultimate goals. If you set your expectations too high, or try to make too many changes at once, you will undoubtedly fail.

For example, suppose one of your weaknesses is an ice cream sundae every night before bedtime. We're hopeful that you now know that eating a high-fat, high-calorie food right before bed is particularly inadvisable both because it can cause GERD and because such snacks can contribute to weight gain. You may also be accustomed to drinking three of four cups of coffee or several cans of soda. The best way to approach changing any of these habits is to cut one "vice" at a time, replacing it with an alternative. Once you've formed this good habit, you can move on to the next. You can stop the nightly ice cream and say to yourself, "I'll treat myself and have that once a week only and have it immediately following my dinner instead of right before I go to bed." The other nights you may want to make a protein shake or eat a protein bar, instead.

After a while you will get used to it and no longer even want to eat the ice cream, particularly if you lose a few pounds in the process and you feel and look better! Then you can tackle the coffee or soda issue. You may want to tell yourself you'll have one can of soda a day, or even none, but in exchange, you'll drink bottled water instead. After a while, you won't want the soda (it makes you thirsty anyway) and you'll feel better about drinking the water. After you've taken off a few more pounds, you'll realize that all you need to do is learn new habits by replacing the old, unhealthy ones with new healthy ones. You will undoubtedly feel better about yourself, your body and your reflux!

RULE 5: *Don't try to achieve all your dietary goals at once.* Chances are it took at least a few years to develop bad habits and/or extra pounds you may have. Fad diets not only don't work, they may be especially harmful to GERD sufferers because they are generally unbalanced and may contain foods that are harmful to your stomach and esophagus. Also, the ability to change dietary habits and/or lose weight depends on age, gender, and your general health. Your doctor can help you create the diet plan that is most likely to work for you.

RULE 6: At least until you get used to eating differently, whenever possible, *prepare your own food.* It is the only way you'll know for sure what you're eating. It's also less expensive and (potentially) a whole lot healthier! We recommend eating organic foods as much as possible, because they don't contain chemical additives or preservatives.

RULE 7: Empty your refrigerator and cupboards of junk food and fatty foods. Load up on healthy, low-fat snacks like fresh fruit and vegetables (except, of course, for those citrus fruits that may cause GERD symptoms). If it's not in your cupboards or refrigerator, you're much less likely to eat it. Don't temp yourself.

RULE 8: *When you are eating, try not to do anything else.* If you are watching television or reading the paper while you eat, it is much easier to eat too fast or eat too much, even if you are full.

RULE 9: *Take small bites.* Unfortunately, because Americans eat so frequently on the run, we eat much too quickly. As a result, many digestive problems are caused not so much by what food we eat but by the way we eat it. Our digestive system is designed to process our food in a specific sequence. When we skip a step, like sending large quantities of underchewed food to our stomachs too fast, often we can experience reflux, particularly if we have any diseases such as diabetes or scleroderma, which can predispose us to reflux. Eat slowly and enjoy your food.

RULE 10: *Chew each bite thoroughly.* Digestion starts in the mouth, not the stomach. Since saliva contains the first of the digestive enzymes, it starts the process, followed by the action of your teeth and tongue to reduce food to small particles. So give it a chance to work. It is also important for the saliva to moisten the food so that it can proceed smoothly down the esophagus. This is particularly important in patients with strictures or esophagitis from reflux. Large foods can also get stuck and cause harm to your esophagus.

RULE 11: *Put your eating utensils down between bites.* If you have ever been on a weight loss diet, you have probably heard this suggestion before. The idea behind this suggestion is both to slow down your eating and to get you to chew your food more thoroughly.

RULE 12: *Avoid drinking excessive amounts of carbonated beverages with your meals*, or better yet, avoid drinking carbonated beverages altogether.

Drinking them is not a good idea because carbonated beverages cause gas to form in the stomach and can make what may already be a bad situation much, much worse.

That may seem like a pretty big list of don'ts. But if you try to be aware of them, you should soon see positive results. Sometimes even changing a few things about the way you eat can make a big difference in the amount and severity of GERD you will experience. If your GERD is particularly severe, you should do your best to follow the advice in this chapter as strictly as possible.

## A Recommended Daily Menu

If you have been suffering from GERD for some time, by the time you see a doctor, you may have tried a wide variety of remedies and diets. And all this experimentation may have left you feeling confused about what to do. Although a new diet is something that you and your doctor will need to develop together to meet your individual situation, here are some general suggestions.

### Breakfast

CEREAL Most dry breakfast cereal is a good thing to eat in the morning. Many commercially prepared cereals are fortified with many of the vitamins you need and cereal also tends to contain both fiber and a portion of the amount of whole grains you should have. However, if you need to lose weight, be aware that there is a big difference in the amount of calories and fat in the many, many kinds of cereal on the market. A cup of Product 19®, for example has 100 calories and no grams of fat, while just 3/4 cup of Cracklin Oat Bran® has 190 calories and 7 grams of fat.

Most cooked cereals are a good nutritional choice, as well, although if they are flavored with "something," that something may add calories and fat.

To achieve a balanced diet, be sure to measure your cereal before putting it in the bowl and compare it to the "serving size" on the box.

Also be sure to count the fats, carbohydrates and protein in the milk you add.

Fortunately, milk is widely available in a variety of forms, to meet the dietary needs of people of all ages. Whole milk contains significantly more fat than 2%, 1% , or skim milk. Many people have little trouble stepping down from 2% milk and then later, to 1% milk and finally skim milk as soon as they see the difference in the numbers of calories and fat consumed just this one change can make

EGGS. Eggs are not extraordinarily high in calories, nor do they seem to cause problems for people with GERD. A medium-sized egg has about 70 calories. Egg yolks, however are fairly high in fat (about 4 grams per egg) and are not recommended for people who tend to have high cholesterol.

Where most people pick up the calories and fat that can make eggs hard to digest, however, is in how the eggs are prepared. While a single hard boiled egg has no more calories than a raw one, a two-egg serving of eggs Benedict on an English muffin (primarily because of the hollandaise sauce) has 860 calories and 56 grams of fat. When possible, either hard boil eggs or prepare them with a non-fat cooking spray.

If you like the taste of eggs for breakfast every day, you might try some of the egg substitutes now available, but as with regular eggs, how you prepare them is still an important consideration. Another good option is egg white meals. While high in protein, they are virtually fat free. You can add a yolk the mix if you want a yellow omelet or scrambled eggs and it will taste great. I typically make a 4 to 6 egg white dish for breakfast in the morning and I'll add 1 yolk per 6 whites. The fat is significantly less and it tastes great. It's also a very inexpensive breakfast and easy to prepare. You can add mushrooms, onions and herbs for more flavor while reducing the likelihood of GERD and the cutting down on fat.

MEAT. Many people still enjoy meat with breakfast. But since meat is a high fat food and is more difficult to digest than cereals and breads, meat should be eaten in moderation. Two strips of bacon, well drained, have about 70 calories and 5 grams of fat. Two ounces of lean ham have about 100 calories and 3 grams of fat. A good alternative is turkey bacon or other lower fat substitutes. Bacon does taste great so if you have to have it, try to minimize it. My overall recommendation, though, would be to stop eating bacon if you have GERD.

BREAD. Most Americans eat some sort of bread for breakfast and it, like cereal, is not a bad choice since bread contains whole grains and, if purchased commercially, usually has vitamins and minerals added to it. In choosing bread, however, it is very important to read the label on the package, since people suffering from GERD often need to watch their fat intake. Remember, that bread is also high calorie so too much of it can make you put on weight. Remember that fat content alone is not the only with regard to a healthy diet! Too many calories a day amounts to pounds gained!

There is a huge variation in what is contained in our breakfast bread favorites. "Light" bread, for example, contains about 40 calories and 1 or 2 grams of fat per slice, while a glazed donut contains about 250 calories and 12 grams of fat. What can really fool you are bagels. They may look pretty healthy, but the average bagel has just about the same number of calories as a donut. What is different, of course, is the fat, since bagels are boiled, not deep fried. A 250-calorie bagel has only 1 or 2 grams of fat, the same as the light bread. Muffins are also a popular breakfast choice. But, again, if you are concerned about calories and fat, you need to read labels carefully. Weight Watchers low fat muffins only have 175 calories and 3 grams of fat, but a 4 ounce Otis Spunkmeyer banana muffin has 480 calories and 24 grams of fat.

Additionally, it is important to watch what you put on the bread you eat. One ounce of cream cheese adds 80 calories and 8 grams of fat. A teaspoon of butter adds 35 calories and 4 grams of fat (margarine is about the same), a teaspoon of honey adds 22 calories and a tablespoon of fruit jelly adds about 18 calories, but there is virtually no fat in jelly or honey.

As convenient as they might be, beware of toaster pastries. They are usually high in both calories and fat.

BEVERAGES Finding a breakfast beverage can be a challenge for those suffering from GERD. All of the traditional American favorites—coffee, tea and orange juice—are, strictly speaking, off limits. However, many people feel that giving up these foods is really difficult, so you might not try to give them up all at once. Instead try to do without them a few days a week at first. There are many things you might substitute. The juices that seem to cause GERD are mostly citrus, including orange, lime, lemon, and grapefruit. Instead, try apple, cranberry, grape, or better yet, mix those juices together with yogurt or fruits such as bananas and strawberries to create a delicious smoothie (See pages 235 to 251). If you just can't get used to not having a hot beverage for breakfast, consider drinking one of the fruit juices hot. Hot cranberry juice with a little cinnamon added makes a great start to a cold winter day.

YOGURT Yogurt makes an excellent breakfast food. It's now available in dozens of flavors, as well as in regular, low-fat and fat-free products. If you are dieting, be sure to read the label since one container of yogurt can vary from between about 100 calories and one gram of fat to 250 calories and 4 or 5 grams of fat.

## Midmorning Snack

For a mid-morning snack, you might be tempted to go down to your break room vending machine, but unless your place of business is exceptionally health conscious, the vending machine is something you should probably avoid. Most are stocked primarily with candy bars and snack foods like potato chips.

Candy bars are not a good option for several reasons. Most contain chocolate which tends to relax the lower esophageal sphincter muscle (LES) and contribute to incidents of reflux. Also, most candy bars are very high in calories and fat. A regular Hershey Bar has 240 calories and 14 grams of fat. Now, many candy bars are available in several sizes, so you must take that into consideration. For example, a king-sized Hershey Bar has 410 calories and 25 grams of fat. Four ounces of potato chips have 600 calories and 40 grams of fat. Pretzels are a lower fat alternative, but they have about the same number of calories as chips.

We recommend that you bring your own snacks to work. You may not only save money (snack foods are expensive) but you will feel better about yourself if you have a healthy snack. An apple, a banana or a pear, for example, has about 90 calories and no fat at all. A peach has even fewer calories and still no fat. The yogurt we mentioned for breakfast also makes a nice mid-morning snack. Combine your snack with a bottle of flavored water, plain water or a non-citrus fruit juice.

## Lunch

As you try to change your eating habits, it might be a good idea to bring your lunch from home so that you will know exactly what is in the foods you're eating. If you like sandwiches, your most healthy choices are the sliced meats you buy in the deli section of your grocery store. Two 2-ounce slices of deli turkey, chicken, ham or lean beef contain only 1 or 2 grams of fat and about 50 calories. If you combine one of those with lettuce and no-fat mayonnaise or mustard on two slices of light bread, you will have gained only another 70 or 80 calories and no extra fat. If you miss the crunchiness of a tomato in a sandwich, try substituting cucumber slices. Remember, too, to avoid catsup, since it is a tomato product.

Soup is another good choice for lunch. Now there are many dried soups on the market that can quickly be prepared with a cup of boiling water. Many canned soups are now also available in one-serving containers. Soups vary from 60 to about 250 calories per serving, depending on what is in them. If you are going to eat the whole can of soup, be sure to note how many servings it contains and adjust your calorie count accordingly. Be sure to read the label and avoid tomato-based soups. Also, if you are watching your salt intake, be aware that many prepared soups have a high sodium content. Canned soups in particular are typically loaded with fat.

Lunch is also another good time to eat a piece of fruit. If you like something sweet to finish your noon meal, have a peach instead of ice cream or a candy bar.

If it is impossible for you to bring your lunch to work, or if you travel and have to eat in restaurants, whenever possible try to order foods that are not combined with other things. For example, try to avoid entrees that have multiple ingredients combined with sauces, particularly those like pasta dishes that contain tomatoes or tomato products, as well as pastas with rich creamy sauces.

The same goes for sandwiches. While a grilled chicken sandwich may seem like a healthy choice, most restaurants serve these sand-wiches with cheese, mayonnaise and other ingredients that add both calories and fat. A better choice would be a grilled chicken breast with steamed vegetables (although many restaurants cover the steamed vegetables with butter). Salads are a good choices, although, again, most restaurant salads are full of ingredients like cheese and bacon that add calories and tomatoes that are acidic. Also, even with salads, keep in mind what a "serving" is. Many restaurant salads now are very large (although some now offer a "lunch" size). If you are going to have a restaurant salad, you may wish to bring along your own dressing, as, again, dressing can add calories and fat. Most low fat dressings are now available in small packets that are easy to carry with you. A great choice to consider for a relatively healthy and flavorful salad dressing is balsamic vinegar. You can use this alone or with a small amount of oil.

Also, if you are trying to lose weight, beware of the extras that come with your meal, like crackers, chips or French fries. Instead of a carbonated soft drink, order water with a lemon or lime. One lemon or lime wedge in a glass of water typically does not warrant concern for reflux or cause you much trouble. A great alternative for a side dish for your sandwich would be to ask for salad instead of French fries or potato chips. Most restaurants or delis will accommodate this.

## Afternoon Snack

If you've had a piece of fruit for your morning snack, you may want something different for your afternoon snack. While, again, that vending machine may look awfully tempting, resist. It seems like someone in just about every office whips up a batch of microwave popcorn in the middle of the afternoon and the aroma seems to reach everywhere. For you, vegetables like celery and baby carrots dipped in low or no-calorie ranch dressing are a much better choice, since most popcorn is flavored with butter and salt. If you crave something salty, consider some of the new baked chips or low-fat crackers with some low-fat cheese. (Hummus is another alternative, although some hummus may be flavored with tomato sauce. (See pages 235 to 251 for a healthy hummus recipe).

## Dinner

Since you have already had four smaller meals during the day, chances are you will not be as hungry for dinner as if you had either only had breakfast or lunch or you had skipped a meal, which is not a good rule to follow. As you get used to this new way of eating, try not preparing quite as much food as usual.

If you are accustomed to having a glass of wine, a beer or a cocktail before dinner, try substituting flavored water or fruit juice. Alcohol not only adds calories but also stimulates the production of stomach acid which may be an irritant to the lining of your esophagus. It is a bad idea to irritate these areas right before your stomach will be starting to produce the additional acid it will need to digest your dinner. Substitute a glass of fruit juice or a flavored, non-carbonated water, or just plain water.

Since you will likely have more time for your dinner than any other meal, I also recommend that you plan a dinner that can be served in courses rather than all at once. You might start with a salad or soup, than have a main course and a dessert.

Serving meals in courses also allows you to take more time eating, which, in turn, gives your stomach a chance to begin digesting your food at a more leisurely pace. It will also allow you to enjoy your meal more comfortably. Eating foods separately helps you enjoy each food more, since you will be eating it in isolation from other flavors. Furthermore, if you take the time to actually savor each bite, chances are you will eat less.

Although Europeans eat food that we might consider to be much richer than what we eat and drink and more wine than we do, on the whole they have fewer problems with obesity and digestive problems. One reason may be they typically take a longer period of time to eat a meal and the quantity they eat is much less. We'd suggest starting with a salad or soup. Follow that with a main course that consists of a small portion of baked or broiled meat, a starchy food such as a baked potato and at least one green or yellow vegetable, preferably either baked or steamed. If you're game to try eating European, then have your salad. If you grew up enjoying something sweet at the end of the meal, have some low or no-fat pudding or a frozen fruit bar or one of the desserts in the recipe section at the end of this book.

Wine if it is to be consumed, should be done so with great caution. Any alcoholic beverage can induce reflux disease by both relaxing the LES and causing local irritation of the esophageal lining regardless of whether or not food is consumed with the wine. If you drink wine, keep the quantity minimal. Just as it is a good idea to eat food slowly, savoring each bite, so too is wine enjoyed best sipped, rather than gulped down. Although most reflux sufferers have experience symptoms with alcohol intake. Avoidance is the best policy, particularly if the hour is late or near bedtime. Many people who drink excess alcohol at night have nighttime reflux, even those people who don't ordinarily experience GERD.

Beer, in addition to being an alcoholic beverage is also carbonated, so beer is probably an even worse choice of beverage if you have GERD.

## A Better Choice for an All-American Diet

Remember the 'All Too Typical American Diet' in Chapter 7? A more healthful diet looks a bit more like the following

|  | CALORIES | FAT (G) | CARBS (G) | FIBER (G) | PROTEIN (G) |
|---|---|---|---|---|---|
| **BREAKFAST** | | | | | |
| 1 slice low fat bread | 35 | 1 | 9 | 3 | 2 |
| 1 tsp honey | 25 | | 5 | | 0 |
| 1/2 cup granola | 220 | 7.5 | 48 | 3 | 2 |
| 1 cup 2% milk | 121 | 5 | 12 | 0 | 8 |
| 1 cup apple juice | 117 | 0 | 29 | 0 | 0 |
| TOTAL | 518 | 13.5 | 103 | 6 | 12 |
| **MID MORNING SNACK** | | | | | |
| 1 container fat free yogurt | 100 | 0 | 19 | 0 | 13 |
| **LUNCH** | | | | | |
| 1 cup dried chicken noodle soup | 60 | 1.5 | 10 | 0 | |
| 2 slices low fat bread | 70 | 2 | 18 | 6 | 4 |
| 2 oz deli-style chicken | 60 | 2 | 1 | 0 | 10 |
| 1 slice Swiss cheese | 110 | 9 | 1 | | 8 |
| Lettuce | 0 | 0 | 0 | 0 | 0 |
| Fat free mayonnaise | 12 | 0 | 3 | 0 | 0 |
| TOTAL | 312 | 14.5 | 23 | 6 | 23 |
| **AFTERNOON SNACK** | | | | | |
| 1 cup raw carrots | 31 | 1 | 7 | 2 | 1 |
| 1 cup apricot nectar | 140 | 0 | 35 | 0 | 0 |
| TOTAL | 171 | 1 | 42 | 2 | 1 |

| Before dinner | | | | | |
|---|---|---|---|---|---|
| 1 cup cranberry juice | 120 | 0 | 34 | 0 | 0 |

| Dinner | | | | | |
|---|---|---|---|---|---|
| 6 ounces broiled chicken breast | 285 | 6 | 0 | 0 | 55 |
| 1 med. Baked potato | 220 | 0 | 51 | 5 | 5 |
| 2t sour cream | 60 | 6 | 1 | 0 | 0 |
| 1 cup broccoli | 50 | 0 | 5 | 3 | 3 |
| 1 slice low fat bread | 35 | 1 | 9 | 3 | 2 |
| 1 tsp. fat-free jelly | 0 | 0 | 0 | 0 | 0 |
| 1cup strawberries | 45 | 0 | 11 | 3 | 1 |
| 2T fat-free whipped topping | 15 | 0 | 3 | 0 | 0 |
| Total | 710 | 13 | 80 | 14 | 66 |

| Snack | | | | | |
|---|---|---|---|---|---|
| 3 Graham crackers | 105 | 1.5 | 15 | 0 | 0 |
| Daily Total | 2036 | 43.5 | 316 | 28 | 114 |

| Grams times 9 calories for fat, times 4 calories for carbohydrates and protein | | 391.5 | 1264 | | 456 |
|---|---|---|---|---|---|
| Percentages | | 19.2% | 62% | | 22% |

As you can see, this menu would help you achieve the desired number of calories from protein, calories and fat.

| Calories from | 2,000 calories per day | 3,000 calories per day |
|---|---|---|
| Protein | 300–400 | 450–600 |
| Fat | 400–600 | 600–900 |
| Carbohydrates | 1000–1300 | 1500–1950 |

You can also see how eating the foods suggested in the above chart would help you achieve the suggested goal of 15 to 20 percent of calories from protein, 20 to 30 percent from fat and 50 to 65 percent from carbohydrates. The dietary plan also includes the recommended 25 grams of fiber.

Let's compare this day's worth of food with the USDA's Food Guide Pyramid.

| | |
|---|---|
| FATS, SWEETS, OILS | (USE SPARINGLY) |
| MEAT/MEAT SUBSTITUTE | (2 TO 3 SERVINGS PER DAY |
| MILK/MILK SUBSTITUTE | (2 TO 3 SERVINGS PER DAY) |
| FRUIT | (2 TO 4 SERVINGS PER DAY) |
| VEGETABLES | (3 TO 5 SERVINGS PER DAY) |
| BREAD, CEREAL, RICE, PASTA | (6 TO 11 SERVINGS PER DAY; 4 TO 6 FOR WEIGHT LOSS) |

If you consumed our recommended diet, you would have had six servings of bread and cereal, four servings of vegetables, five servings of fruit and six servings of milk and meat. While this menu may be slightly lower in protein than the guidelines recommend, it's not bad. Plus, if you were trying to lose some weight, you will notice that this menu is comparatively low in fat.

Changing any life-long habit, particularly one that is as familiar as eating is often not an easy task. But I think you will find that if you will just make these few alterations, you can begin to see a noticeable difference both in the way your feel and the way you look.

# 9

# EXERCISE
## *Making the Right Choices*

J UST ABOUT EVERY PATIENT ASKS HIS OR HER doctor about exercise. Athletic patients are concerned about whether or not exercise causes their GERD; sedentary patients ask whether their lack of exercise makes them prone to GERD.

In general, exercise is an excellent way to relieve stress and anxiety, to lose weight, and allow patients to experience an overall sense of well-being once a routine is achieved. Almost everyone finds that they feel and look better when they exercise regularly.

Whether you're an elite athlete or are just considering an exercise program, there are some facts you should know about the relationship between exercise and GERD. The first, and perhaps most important fact is that there are some types of exercises all GERD sufferers should avoid. Even those that might be beneficial to your overall health may not be appropriate for you as a GERD sufferer. They generally include:

Exercises that put a lot of strain on the abdominal muscles, such as strenuous weight lifting, gymnastics, rock climbing, competitive cycling, wrestling, kick boxing, calisthenics and sometimes even shoveling snow.

Exercises that cause a lot of repeated up and down motion, such as vigorous running, high impact aerobics, or jumping rope.

Exercises that require strenuous movement for a long period of time or bursts of sudden speed, such as running (particularly sprinting), long distance swimming or cycling, and vigorous team sports such as football, basketball, rugby, or racquetball.

If you currently engage in any of these exercises, you may want to consider replacing them with less strenuous activity. Although you may not receive the same benefits (either physical or psychological) from less strenuous exercise, you should find that your problems with GERD have greatly decreased. Finding a happy medium is important for achieving success in your exercise regimen as well achieving symptom reduction from GERD.

Recommending exercise to GERD patients is not a cut and dried affair. What is best for one patient must take into account the patient's build and constitution, functional status and interest level, and the baseline exercise regimen the patient is following when he or she arrives at the doctor's office.

## The Downside of Exercise

Unfortunately, exercise, at least some forms of exercise, can cause a variety of unpleasant results including abdominal pain, diarrhea, gastrointestinal bleeding, and GERD. In general, runners seem most troubled by lower bowel symptoms, while weight lifters and cyclists are more commonly troubled by heartburn.

If the heart rate goes up, which is nearly always the case with physical exertion, the amount of blood flow seems to decrease, particularly in organs such as the stomach. If physical exertion occurs following a meal, the result can be a slowing of gastric emptying with a feeling of nausea, and sometimes the urge to vomit or actual vomiting. Significant gastro-esophageal reflux can also be a result.

The digestive system characteristically works better when the body is at rest. During vigorous exercise, digestion slows down and the stomach cannot empty as quickly as it does when you are sitting at your desk or taking a leisurely stroll. When digestion slows down gastric emptying is slowed, as it does with fatty meals and the likelihood of an episode of GERD increases. What your mother told you about not swimming until an hour after lunch does have a physiological justification, after all.

Aerophagia, or taking in large gulps of air can be another problem caused by participation in vigorous sports. Running very fast, jogging, swimming, or cycling for a long time or playing sports that require sudden bursts of speed tends to cause athletes to take in large gulps of air, which puts pressure on the LES. When sudden or intense pressure is applied to the LES, the "valve" can then open up allowing air to escape, causing belching as well as reflux of gastric contents. Carbonated beverages might have a similar effect since the expanding gas stretches the lining of the stomach as well.

While exercising, athletes also often take in liquid in large swallows. The immediate effect of all this liquid flowing down the esophagus and hitting the LES can be nausea or vomiting. The longer-term effect may be GERD.

There is also some evidence to suggest that an intense amount of exercise affects the motility (i.e. movement) of the muscles in the intestines, pushing the food along at a faster than average pace. The result of this can be diarrhea, or even intestinal bleeding (although this is seen very rarely).

Colonic transit time (the time it takes for food and digested material to flow through the colon) can also be accelerated during extreme exercise. The release of hormones (endorphins) that some extreme athletes experience (sometimes known as "runner's high") may also affect the digestive process by either inducing GERD or causing diarrhea. Vigorous exercise also tends to lower the pressure of the LES, allowing the undigested food to reflux up into the esophagus.

While many athletes who are in superb physical shape experience GERD or one of several other gastrointestinal complaints, the likelihood of trouble tends to be even more pronounced in athletes who are overweight or out of condition. In these cases, the problem may be compounded by increased pressure on the stomach from excess fat around the middle. Therefore, extreme exercise can cause significant negative effects in both fit and not-so-fit athletes. Moderate or low level exercise, at less risk of causing GERD, is also less likely to result in pronounced symptoms.

Finally, although Lycra and Spandex do make fairly impressive fashion statements, garments that fit very tightly around the waist and upper torso are well known causes for gastro-esophageal reflux disease. These do so by applying pressure upon the abdomen (specifically the diaphragm), especially in the case of athletes like cyclists who bend forward for long periods of time.

## The Upside of Exercise

While some types of exercise, particularly extreme types of sports or endurance sports can cause episodes of GERD, at least a moderate amount of exercise will not only relieve your symptoms, but can greatly improve your overall health, as well. Exercise, if performed cautiously at a low to moderate level will almost always be beneficial.

## Exercises for GERD Patients

Fortunately, with the exception of extremely vigorous sports or those that require considerable endurance, most forms of exercise, in moderation, are not only appropriate for GERD sufferers, but also greatly beneficial. Weight lifting (excluding profoundly heavy weights or power lifting), fast paced walking or low level jogging are all excellent habits to develop. Lower impact exercises performed on a regular basis with increasing muscle strength can allow you to lose weight and add to an overall sense of well-being.

The kind of exercise that is right for you depends on several factors:

WHAT EXERCISES YOU CURRENTLY PARTICIPATE IN. If you are now participating in extremely vigorous or endurance sports and you have no symptoms of GERD while performing this type of exercise, continue with your usual regimen. If you are a highly competitive person, moderation may be difficult. The best advice is to follow your symptoms. If you are a competitive athlete and your reflux is unbearable or highly symptomatic, it certainly would not seem to benefit you to continue years of training at this level. Instead, you may need to consider the possibility of lessening either the pace or the intensity of your workout. In general, GERD should be worse during extreme exercise, but it can certainly occur at any time, even when you are not exercising. Athletes with GERD experience a variety of symptoms, but a general rule is that extreme running and heavy lifting cause worsening symptoms.

Having said this, however, if you're an elite athlete, you'll have no long-term effects if symptoms only occur in competition. If they occur at every practice, however, then you'll probably have to take long term medicines or possibly turn to surgery (see page 182) to relieve the symptoms. In any event, if you are a competitive athlete with significant symptoms of reflux, you should certainly consult a gastroenterologist to discuss the options available to you. If you have minimal to no reflux while vigorously exercising, there is no reason to stop.

WHAT EXERCISES YOU ENJOY. If you're not currently exercising, you should probably first try several forms of low-impact exercise such as walking, swimming, cycling, golf or bowling. Choose those you like best and that don't trigger symptoms. While exercise is good for you, it shouldn't be a punishment. All forms of exercise, including Yoga, are a good alternative for most people. Any exercise you chose, however, has the potential to induce GERD, including Yoga (because of the body contortions required), but you'll only know if you try it. Do something you enjoy.

YOUR AGE. Fortunately, doctors have now come to recognize that exercise should be a lifelong activity. But what is appropriate for our bodies at age 16 may not be as good for us when we're 85. While some things like walking or swimming are good for you no matter how old or young you are, remember that exercise should be something that helps you, not injures you. If you are just starting an exercise program, check with your doctor about what type of exercise would be the most appropriate for someone your age and in your current physical condition.

YOUR CURRENT STATE OF HEALTH. If you have other medical problems, such as heart disease, diabetes or any other medical condition, you should consult your physician prior to embarking on an exercise plan, particularly if it is a rigorous one.

Other health concerns. Similarly, you need to be aware of what effect starting an exercise program might have on your body if you are a smoker or you are overweight, if you have or had cancer, prior surgery, if you have peripheral vascular disease or any other chronic condition.

Where you live. Many people live in a climate where they can do essentially the same kind of exercise year-round. Others live in places where the climate changes dramatically from season to season. Although it is certainly possible to do all of your exercise indoors at a gym, my advice is to do at least some of it outdoors and to vary what you do to match the seasons. This will make it more fun and help to ensure compliance with your exercise regimen. If you enjoy your surroundings and your overall experience, it will undoubtedly serve you well in the long run.

Whether you need to lose weight. As we all know, the older we get the harder it seems to be to lose weight. One reason for that (in addition to the frequent failure of fad diets) is that we don't combine our diet with exercise. If you don't need to lose weight, you may not need more than 30 minutes of exercise three times a week. But if weight loss is a goal, you need to create an exercise program that will help you take off the pounds that will be hard to eliminate by a diet alone.

YOUR DAILY SCHEDULE. One of the many excuses people give me for not exercising is that they just don't have time. While it is true that most of us have far busier schedules than we perhaps should, exercise must be made a priority in your day-to-day planning. You will find that exercise will not only help you maintain a healthy weight, but will also give you more energy for the other activities in your life.

WHAT IS PRACTICAL FOR YOU. At the same time, make sure that the exercise program you choose will be practical, that is physically available to you. Ask your doctor about facilities in your community that provide the best exercise options for you.

HOW DISCIPLINED YOU ARE. Some people have no problem at all rolling out of bed at 5:00 a.m. three days a week and going across town to a gym before work. But if that doesn't sound like you, design an exercise program that you know you will actually do. Use at least a couple of lunch hours a week to take a brisk walk and one longer period on the weekend to do something else you enjoy. With regard to time spent, a healthy aerobic exercise regimen even three times a week can significantly contribute to better health and wellbeing. You should not consider this impossible. For many, it can mean substituting exercise time for watching morning or early evening television. Or, better yet, if you purchase a treadmill or stationary bike, you can watch your favorite programs and exercise at the same time.

WHAT YOU CAN AFFORD. As you might imagine, there is literally no end to how much money you can spend on exercise equipment or memberships in fancy health clubs. But none of these reasons are adequate to argue for a lack of ability to perform exercise. Many businesses now have workout facilities available to employees or offer discounts to employees at area gyms. Most communities also have a YMCA, YWCA, community center or school that has all the facilities you need at a reasonable price. And, of course, it costs nothing at all to take a walk in the park.

## Before Beginning

Even if you are in perfect health, it is always advisable to consult your doctor before you begin an exercise program of any kind. You need to make sure that your heart is healthy and that there are no other physical limitations that would be exacerbated by specific types of exercise. If you are a GERD sufferer, you should avoid exercise that strains the abdominal muscles or requires considerable endurance.

## Getting Started

If you are not currently exercising at all, start slowly. For example, if you have decided that you might enjoy walking, start by walking 10 to 15 minutes every other day. After a week or two, increase that time to 30 minutes and then after another two weeks or so, increase to 45 minutes and then to an hour. The same regimen might apply to cycling or to swimming. After achieving this goal, try to increase the interval to daily exercise if possible. If you live in a very hot or cold climate, or a climate where the weather changes frequently, you might consider joining the local Y, a gym or a health club where you could use indoor equipment such as treadmills or stationary bicycles when the weather is inclement. Many enclosed shopping malls now also allow you to come in before the mall opens and walk. On the other hand, if you live in an area where the climate changes, you may well find the variety of exercise options provided by warm and cold weather will make your exercise program more interesting and, thus, make you more likely to keep doing it. And, of course, you can take a brisk walk outdoors in just about any weather.

## How Much is Enough?

If you do not need to lose weight, most studies have shown that 30 minutes to an hour, three times a week is sufficient for cardiac fitness. If you do need to lose weight, however, you will probably need to increase the amount of exercise you do now so that you can burn up more calories. Walking a mile, for example, burns up about 150 calories, while walking four miles burns up more than 500.

The study by the Institute of Medicine of the National Academy of Science released in September 2002 increased the traditional 30-minute, three times a week recommendation to one hour a day. While this amount of exercise might be desirable, admittedly, for many people that amount may be impractical, especially since for most people getting in a daily exercise session also involves changing clothes, showering and so on.

One hour a day of aerobic exercise would be an overall excellent accomplishment. But if you aren't able to commit that much time, don't give up on exercising. Performing aerobic exercise for 20 minutes three times a week also greatly improves your overall health and cardiovascular status.

Some people are more limited than others in the amount of exercise they can perform, but no one should ever allow themselves to become sedentary. A sedentary lifestyle is bad for your heart and it will inevitably result in weight gain. This lifestyle is also a significant contributor to episodes of GERD.

## Weight Training

Weight training was once considered a program designed solely to enhance the development of large muscles in both men and women. In more recent years, we have come to understand that developing and maintaining muscle tone is a good idea for just about everybody of every age from toddlers to the very old. One of the main benefits of weight training is to not only enhance muscle strength, but also bone strength. For these reasons, weight training is a staple in any exercise program.

You should, however, note that there are some limitations for patients with GERD. If you have GERD, you should plan your work-out so that you avoid excess pressure on your abdominal muscles. Fortunately, most fitness facilities now have many different kinds of machines that focus and isolate specific muscle groups without applying undue stress on others. We also recommend that, at least at first, you seek the guidance of a personal trainer who also has knowledge in or is a professional in exercise physiology to help you plan your workout routine. These professionals will not only be able to prescribe the exercises that are most appropriate for you, but will supervise your workout to make sure you both avoid hurting yourself and that you progress to heavier weights and more repetitions in a healthy and productive way.

## Other Hints to Keep in Mind

EXERCISE WITH A FRIEND.  Even if you greatly enjoy exercise, you will generally find that time will pass more quickly if you have someone to talk to and someone to inspire you to exercise on a regular schedule.

VARY YOUR EXERCISE ROUTINE. No matter how good for you it is, exercise, like everything else can soon become monotonous. And when this happens, unfortunately, you will find that it is easy to find excuses not to do it. Find a variety of ways to achieve the same thing. If you enjoy walking, walk a different route each day. On weekends make it a point to visit different parts of town or explore new neighborhoods. If you find that you are getting tired of walking, try swimming or cycling or ice skating. Or, better yet, do different types of exercises on different days of the week.

SET GOALS. One of the many advantages of exercise is that in general the more faithful you are to your exercise program, the better you will get at it. Once you achieve a comfort level, you will want to do more of that type of exercise. You'll notice that your endurance will improve and with time, you will likely push yourself a little bit harder. While, again, you will want to avoid extremely vigorous exercise or endurance sports, you should push yourself to a limit that you find acceptable. With regard to GERD, many patients know their limitations by recognizing when and if symptoms are worsened. If you enjoy walking, enter a few charity walkathons. If you like to play golf, entering a tournament will also help to keep you active as well as encourage a continued interest in the sport.

# 10

# MEDICATION FOR GERD
## *Learning About the Options*

I N THIS CHAPTER WE DISCUSS THE MEDICATIONS that have been specifically formulated to help GERD sufferers. The prevalence of heartburn in the United States has resulted in the development of different medicines to deal with this condition.

The most recent medications developed are proton pump inhibitors, which are so successful in treating GERD and its complications that several pharmaceutical companies have now produced variations of this drug class in an attempt to maximize benefit and minimize adverse effects and drug interactions.

Although these new drugs are helpful to GERD sufferers, they are much stronger agents than earlier ones and not all patients with GERD need them. Before deciding to try any of these medications, it is important to understand what medications are available for GERD and what makes each different from one another.

There are three major reasons for this. First, you may be taking one or a combination of these medications for a long period of time. It is important to know as much about each of the available agents to choose the most appropriate medicine for you.

Second, the chemicals in each particular medication may cause uncomfortable side effects. Knowing the differences among all of the medicines will help you and your physician determine the best medication or combination of medications. That can mean choosing the medication that works best for you with the fewest side effects and greatest safety profile. For example, patients with kidney disease must be particularly careful with some reflux medicines since some may contain elements that can be harmful in high quantities. Although most antacid formulations are usually well tolerated, it is important to check with a pharmacist or doctor for any potential toxicity of these drugs.

Third, GERD symptoms can be the result of a variety of different physiologic processes. It is important, therefore, to choose the medicine that most effectively targets the cause of those symptoms specific to you.

The availability of so many different medications is good news for GERD sufferers because it is likely that at least one will be effective, On the other hand, the availability of a many products can also make choosing the right one difficult. Before asking for prescription medication for the symptoms of GERD, changes in lifestyle and diet should be attempted to deal with frequent episodes of reflux. Those changes may significantly reduce the symptoms of heartburn.

In this chapter we'll discuss how the drugs prescribed for GERD work and how to take them for the greatest symptom relief and fewest side effects. This chapter also describes the differences among these drugs, their active ingredients, and the best way to take them. This chapter can also act as a guide to use before and after consulting with a physician.

## Available Medications

Drugs designed to treat acid reflux fall into five main classifications:

1. *Antacids*—over the counter and prescription

2. *Sucralfate*—prescription only
3. *H-2 blockers*—prescription and over the counter
4. *Pro-motility agents*—prescription
5. *Proton pump inhibitors*—prescription and over the counter

## *Antacids*

Over-the-counter antacids are the medications most frequently used to treat acid reflux. Since acid reflux is such a common problem, it is not surprising that antacids are one of the most commonly taken of all pharmaceutical agents. Because of the proliferation of these drugs, they are widely available without a prescription in convenience stores, grocery stores, and pharmacies throughout the United States and the world. Although H2 blockers and proton pump inhibitors are also considered antacid agents (because they specifically target and inhibit the acid-secreting cells in the stomach), they're discussed in a later section. This section concentrates primarily on the over-the-counter antacids that are not H2 blockers.

How Do Antacids Work? Antacids work by neutralizing acid in the stomach. Acidity (and its opposite, alkalinity) is measured on a 14-point "pH" scale. Something that is absolutely neutral from an acidity/alkalinity perspective has a pH of 7. Any substance with a pH lower than 7 on this scale is an acid and anything higher than a pH of 7 is an alkaline (a base). The lower the number it has on the pH scale, the more acidic the substance. The higher the number it has on the pH scale the more alkaline the substance.

When food enters your mouth and you begin to chew it into small enough portions to swallow, your saliva (which is an alkaline substance) moistens the food and begins to break down starches. In the stomach, acid is produced to chemically break the food down into the nutrients that can be later absorbed by your intestines and provide you with the nourishment you need to stay alive.

In the stomach, food is broken down and most bacteria are killed. Stomach acid, or more specifically, hydrochloric acid, has a pH of 1 or 2—it is an extremely acidic substance. However, it does not damage the stomach because the stomach lining is designed to withstand the effects of this acid for prolonged periods of time with no injury to the gastric mucosa, or lining. High acid states in the stomach persist for the three to four hours that food generally remains in there.

Anywhere outside the stomach, however, prolonged or even brief exposure of acid at this pH level can be extremely corrosive; as corrosive as battery acid in a car. Fortunately, a little acid refluxed into the esophagus, which occurs in just about everyone at one time or another, will probably do little or no harm as long as the acidity doesn't regularly reach 4.0 or less on the pH scale. More than occasional reflux, on the other hand, can be both painful and damaging.

The goal of antacids, which are weak bases, is to combine with the hydrochloric acid in the stomach to produce a salt and water, product of which has a pH greater than 4.0, to neutralize the gastric acidity. If acid with a pH of less than 4.0 is refluxed into the esophagus on a frequent basis, it can cause serious injury to the esophageal tissue. This recurrent injury to the esophagus can lead to esophagitis, its associated symptoms of GERD, the potential for Barrett's esophagus (see Chapter 16), esophageal strictures, and, less likely, esophageal cancer.

If the acid reflux is just an occasional problem, an antacid taken before a meal will usually keep the acid in the stomach at an acceptable pH level and the refluxant (refluxed acid) will be less likely to irritate the esophagus. When the stomach is empty, little acid is produced. Once the acid that was in the stomach is neutralized and no more is produced, pain should abate and there should be little acid available to reflux into the esophagus.

*Note:* While most antacids work by neutralizing acids, bismuth subsalicylate works a bit differently. It stimulates the passage of fluid and electrolytes across the wall of the intestinal tract and can also diminish or halt the toxicity and activity of some bacteria. It may also have the capacity to decrease intestinal inflammation.

WHAT ARE THE LIMITATIONS OF ANTACIDS? The major limitation of antacids is that they work for only a short period of time (usually 60 to 90 minutes depending on the compound or agent used) and only long enough to neutralize the acid that has already been produced to digest whatever is in the stomach. As soon as more food reaches the stomach, however, it begins to produce acid again. Patients who have persistent heartburn and GERD and need to use over-the-counter antacids frequently to counteract acidic symptoms need to consult a physician. Frequent use of antacids is a good indication that the severity of the reflux is too great to be alleviated by over-the-counter medications. A more potent (probably prescription) antacid may be needed.

ACTIVE INGREDIENTS IN ANTACIDS. If every person were physically identical, the formulation of an effective antacid would be a much simpler task. Realistically, however, human beings are quite diverse and have very different metabolic capabilities and extremely varied sensitivities to various agents. Medications, therefore, are developed based on the different metabolic capabilities of each individual. The fact that human beings vary greatly in the way they metabolize enzymes, create and utilize important cells in the body, and by the way their various organs (gastrointestinal tract, liver, and kidneys) break down, absorb, and secrete the chemicals that comprise medications taken by mouth, must also be considered.

Because of this complexity, all pharmaceutical agents or drugs must be critically examined for safety and tolerance. To be approved, drugs must also be designed to be effective in the majority of individuals and must provide the greatest benefit and the lowest risk. Even though all of the agents discussed in this chapter have been FDA approved, all active ingredients in each drug must still be examined with great scrutiny, since each may have profoundly different effects in different individuals.

An example of a physiologic difference among individuals is how acid is secreted. Some patients (hypersecretors) produce an overabundance of gastric acid. At the other end of the spectrum are patients who do not produce enough gastric acid (hyposecretors).

Additionally, everyone absorbs medications in a slightly different way. Some patients may also be taking medications for other illnesses. Those medications can interact with antacids to either limit the effectiveness of the other medications or cause the patient to experience unpleasant side effects. Because of these differences, many different pharmacologic approaches to acid neutralization and inhibition are now available.

The following are the most common ingredients used in over-the-counter antacids. Some contain one of these ingredients, others a combination of them:

- *Aluminum hydroxide (AL(OH3))*
- *Calcium carbonate (CaCO3)*
- *Bismuth subsalicylate (C7H5Bi04)*
- *Magnesium hydroxide (Mg(OH2))*
- *Sodium bicarbonate (NaHCO3)*

The widely available antacids that contain one or more of these ingredients are listed in more detail in charts later in this chapter.

**WHAT ARE THE COMMON SIDE EFFECTS OF ANTACIDS?** Fortunately, because acid reflux is such a common problem, antacids are among the safest medicines available and are free of side effects for most people. Side effects from antacids vary depending on individuals and other medications they may be taking at the time. Those who experience side effects most commonly suffer from changes in bowel functions, such as diarrhea, constipation, or flatulence.

Although reactions to any drug may vary from person to person, generally those medications that contain aluminum or calcium are the likeliest to cause constipation; those that contain magnesium are the likeliest to cause diarrhea. Some products combine these ingredients, which essentially cancels them out, to forestall unpleasant side effects.

In general, people with kidney problems should probably not take antacids of any kind before consulting their doctor because taking antacids can sometimes cause a condition known as alkalosis. In other people, side effects may occur if substances such as salt, sugar, or aspirin, are added to a particular medication. As with all medications, always carefully read the product label on the package and check with your doctor or pharmacist if you have any questions about potential drug interactions or side effects.

Some side effects, such as constipation and diarrhea, are fairly obvious. Other more serious side effects, such as stomach or intestinal bleeding, can often be more difficult to recognize. In general, any sign of blood in the stool or the presence of vomiting is a danger sign and should be brought to the immediate attention of a physician.


WHAT SHOULD YOU KNOW ABOUT DRUG INTERACTIONS? All drugs affect the body. When some drugs are taken at the same time as others, the result can be a chemical reaction that causes unpleasant side effects. Some side effects can be quite serious. Sometimes drugs can also react with certain foods or can be dangerous for people with specific medical conditions. Before taking any drug, whether it is prescription or over-the-counter, you should consult your doctor, pharmacist, or other health care professional. It is important for you to know that what you are taking will not interact in an unpleasant or dangerous way with your other medications.

Remember that alcohol is a drug, as are vitamins, herbal remedies, and supplements. Be sure to tell your doctor if you regularly use any of these products.

WARNINGS ABOUT TAKING ANTACIDS. Although most antacids currently on the market are safe for the vast majority of people, some antacids may not be recommended for people with specific conditions or under certain circumstances.

Some of the warnings listed below are commonly found on the packages of antacid preparations. Some of these warnings are also often seen on the packaging of many other medications, as well. Therefore, many of these warnings are not specific to antacids. Some of the warnings include:

1.  *If you are pregnant* or nursing a baby, you should always consult your doctor before taking this medication.

2.  *If you consume any alcoholic beverages* (or sometimes a specific number of alcoholic beverages) daily, you should not take this medication.

3.  Generally, *you should not give these medications to children under the age of 12* unless under the advice and supervision of your doctor or the package label has indicated that the product is safe for young children.

4.  *If your symptoms persist for more than 10 days to two weeks* while you are using the medication, you should stop taking it and consult your doctor. Persistent symptoms may indicate that you have a more serious problem than occasional acid reflux.

5.  If, when taking this medication, *you begin to experience any prolonged side effects* such as headache, bleeding, constipation, or diarrhea, you should probably discontinue use of the medication and consult your doctor or other health care professional.

6.  *If you are taking any prescription medications,* you should consult your physician before taking these products to make sure that you will not experience adverse drug interactions.

7.  *If you are taking herbal medications,* you should also consult your doctor before taking these products to make sure you will not experience adverse drug interactions.

8. *Keep these and all medicines out of the reach of children.*
9. *Do not use any product if the safety seals have been broken* or it appears the package has been tampered with in any way.

Any special or specific warnings for any of the drugs will be indicated within the charts listed below.

HOW DO I CHOOSE THE BEST ANTACID FOR ME? Some antacids contain just one of the chemicals known to neutralize stomach acid. Others contain combinations of these chemicals along with other drugs, such as aspirin, as well as additives like colorings and flavorings.

The charts below will help you select the one that works best for you and those that cause the fewest side effects. Again, before taking any of these medications, please read the labels carefully and consult with your doctor or pharmacist to be sure the drug you choose will not interact with any other medications you may be taking and that it does not contain substances to which you are allergic.

Please note that the charts that follow include only brand name products that are commonly available at groceries, pharmacies, and on-line mail order sites throughout the United States. The list may not include all products available in your area. Many of these products are also available as store brands. These store-branded products may or may not be exact duplicates of a name brand product and may or may not be less expensive. Some of the products listed here are sold under other trade names in Canada and other countries.

Before using any of these antacids, carefully read the labels on the packaging and within the package inserts. If you have any questions about the product, be sure to consult your doctor, pharmacist, or other health care professional.

SOME HINTS ON TAKING ANTACIDS. When taking chewable tablets, it is generally a good idea to follow the tablets with a glass of water. Many liquid antacids taste better if they are refrigerated. Some antacids are best taken before eating, while others are to be taken after or between meals.

Be sure to read the directions on the package carefully before taking any medication. The dosage specified is the one that has been proved to be the most effective and safest in the majority of patients studied. Generally you should not exceed that amount unless directed by your doctor. The administration and timing of each medication is also important, since many of the different medicines are metabolized in different ways.

If your symptoms persist after two weeks or if you find that you are taking over-the-counter medicines very frequently or multiple times a day, you should consult your doctor to make sure you do not have a more serious problem than occasional acid reflux.

## Sucralfate

Because antacids are effective in neutralizing stomach acid, they are used to prevent damage to the tissue in the esophagus. If damage to these tissues has already occurred, your doctor may recommend sucralfate. This agent may help coat the inflamed or erosive tissue and allow it to heal.

HOW DOES SUCRALFATE WORK? Sucralfate works by coating the surface of an ulcer or protecting tissue from irritation by stomach acid, digestive enzymes, bile salts, and other substances present in the digestive tract. Coating the surface of an ulcer allows the body's normal repair mechanisms to heal the injured tissue without the interference of persistent toxic exposure to gastric acid.

WHAT ARE THE ADVANTAGES OF SUCRALFATE? Sucralfate promotes healing and relieves pain for patients who have either esophageal or gastric ulcers. It also helps protect tissue from damage due to stomach acid and pepsin. Sucralfate is a good choice for immediate relief of symptoms for those who have esophagitis with pain, ulcers higher up in the esophagus, or "kissing" ulcers from pill impaction—that is, ulcers that have spread due to proximity to each other. It may also be recommended for patients who experience significant problems with pain while eating or drinking. The "coating" effect of sucralfate protects ulcers from further injury while also allowing them to heal.

WHAT ARE THE LIMITATIONS OF SUCRALFATE? While sucralfate does protect tissue that has been damaged by acid reflux, it does not treat the cause of acid reflux nor does it neutralize stomach acid.

WHAT ARE THE COMMON SIDE EFFECTS OF SUCRALFATE?
In some patients, a sucralfate may cause constipation.

## Histamine Acid Blockers (H2 blockers)

Throughout most of recorded history, there was little else GERD sufferers could do other than take antacids or go on a diet of extremely bland foods, like Sippy's famous diet, discussed in Chapter 1. When the bland diet didn't help, patients found themselves in a never-ending cycle of pain and antacids while the damage to the esophagus became increasingly more serious, inevitably causing esophagitis in some, and, for the really unfortunate, esophageal ulcerations and even cancer.

In the 1970s, a revolution occurred in the treatment of GERD with the discovery of a family of drugs called histamine receptor antagonists or H2 blockers. Unlike antacids, which relieve GERD symptoms on a short-term basis by neutralizing stomach acid, this new drug was the first to actually significantly decrease the level of production of stomach acid.

HOW DO H2 BLOCKERS WORK? You are probably familiar with the term histamine. Occurring naturally in all animal and vegetable tissues, histamine does four things: dilates capillaries; causes swelling; creates itching; and stimulates gastric secretions. You are probably the most familiar with the first three effects. It is because of the release of these histamines (as a reaction to damage to cell tissue) that an insect bite on your skin swells and itches or urticaria (hives) form when you experience an allergic reaction to something. Drugs used to help alleviate the symptoms of these histamine-induced events are called H1 blockers or antihistamines. Benadryl, Claritin, Coricidin and Visene-A are all popular antihistamines.

Because the fourth effect of histamine occurs in your stomach, it is not as immediately obvious as a mosquito bite or a hive. The release of histamine that causes secretion of stomach acid can also be blocked by a similar class of drugs known as H2 blockers.

**WHAT ARE THE ADVANTAGES OF H2 BLOCKERS?** H2 blockers offer significant relief to many people with GERD. Because these drugs work on only one of the mechanisms in the stomach that secretes acid, some acid will still be secreted and digestion can occur normally. Another major advantage of these H2 blockers is that, if taken correctly, they have few serious side effects, although, because they are powerful drugs, side effects can occur if they are combined with other drugs.

H2 blockers have been shown to heal both gastric and esophageal ulcers, as well as gastritis and symptoms of heartburn. A newer class of drugs, called proton pump inhibitors (PPIs), is an even more potent and effective approach to acid related diseases of the esophagus and stomach. Since not all people need to use these stronger prescription antacid medicines, many people derive great benefit from H2 blockers and do not need to step up to PPIs.

The most commonly prescribed H2 blockers on the market today are Axid, Pepcid, Tagamet, and Zantac. The chart that follows summarizes these drugs, recommended dosages, and possible side effects.

Some prescription H2 blockers are now also available in an over-the-counter form. The only difference between the prescription drugs and the over-the-counter drugs is that, generally, the over-the-counter drugs are in a less concentrated form, often half of the prescription dose.

Doubling up on the over-the-counter form of a medication often approaches the same strength that your doctor would prescribe. The major difference is that the double dosage of an over-the-counter form is more expensive than a single prescription dosage. Also, if you find that you need to take so many over the counter doses for symptom relief, then you should see your doctor for treatment and evaluation. You may be masking a serious underlying problem, and so you should never consider taking more than the recommended dosages of these drugs without first checking with your doctor. Taking more than the recommended dose can also cause undesirable side effects.

## Pro-Motility Agents

In some patients, the cause of acid in the esophagus and heartburn is not only acid refluxing into the esophagus. It can also be poor motility, or movement of the esophageal peristalsis downward. Peristalisis is one of the ways the body clears the esophagus of acid, and so patients with poor motility often have worse reflux than average. Poor motility may occur because the patient has a disease, such as scleroderma, or because the muscles or nerves involving the esophagus do not function properly. Whatever the reason, these patients may benefit from medicines that primarily affect the squeezing of the esophagus, and emptying of the stomach, allowing for better propulsion of food and liquid downward into and out of the stomach.

A major breakthrough in this area was a drug called Propulsid (generic name cisapride). Propulsid was a popular pro-motility drug, but in July 2000, Janssen Pharmaceutica withdrew Propulsid from the United States market because of its side effects (although it is still available to patients who fit strict criteria).

In addition to Propulsid, another medicine is available but its side effects may too limit its use. Reglan's (generic name metoclopramide) effects are mixed at best and the use of this agent may often be complicated by physical and psychological/neurological effects. While many physicians do not use this drug for reflux because of these effects, there is still a role for its use in some, particularly if there is a component of delayed gastric emptying. Currently, newer and less toxic medicines are being studied for use in this area but are not yet available.

## Proton-Pump Inhibitors

In the late 1980s, a new type of drug, called a proton-pump inhibitor (PPI) was developed.

HOW DO PPIS WORK? PPIs, like H2 blockers, work by stopping the production of stomach acid, but PPIs differ from H2 blockers in that they profoundly suppress production of the acid. They do this by restraining a pump in the acid secreting cells of the stomach, called the "proton pump" or "hydrogen pump." This markedly reduces the amount of acid in the stomach and the amount of acid refluxed into the esophagus.

WHAT ARE THE ADVANTAGES OF PPIS? PPIs are more effective and quicker in healing erosive esophagitis than H2 blockers. A further advantage is that most of the drugs made in this class need to be taken only once a day compared to two to four times a day for H2 blockers. In patients where "breakthrough" heartburn occurs at night, PPIs can be taken in the morning on an empty stomach in higher doses or twice a day.

WHAT ARE THE LIMITATIONS OF PPIS? The main disadvantage of PPIs over H2 blockers is that at the time of this printing, they are more expensive than H2 blockers. The chart at the end of this chapter summarizes the most common prescription proton pump inhibitors, their dosages, and potential side effects.

## Summary

The medicines discussed in this chapter represent only a portion of the products now available on the market either under different brand names, store brands, or generic equivalents. Still, they do represent a wide spectrum of the different classifications of drugs used to treat GERD and its symptoms. In Chapter 12, we will discuss some of the herbal remedies that have been used over the centuries, as well as those still used today.

All of the medicines listed in this chapter have been approved for use in the United States by the US Food and Drug Administration. If used according to directions, they should be safe for most sufferers of GERD. Because these medicines work in different ways, however, it is always a good idea to check with your doctor to see which medicines or combinations of medicines are the most likely to work best in your situation. It is also important before taking any new medication to note any potential drug interactions they may have with any of the medicines you are currently taking.

*Antacids That Contain Aluminum Hydroxide*

| Brand Name | Manufacturer | Generic Name | Active Ingredient(s) | Recommended Dosage | Possible Side Effects | Warning |
|---|---|---|---|---|---|---|
| **AlternaGel Antacid Liquid** | Johnson & Johnson-Merck | aluminum hydroxide | Each tsp. contains 600 mg of aluminum hydroxide. | 1-2 tsps. between meals, at bedtime, or as directed by a doctor. | Constipation, chalky taste | Do not take more than 18 tsps. in a 24-hour period or use the maximum dosage for more than 2 weeks. If you have kidney disease, do not use except under the advice of a doctor. |
| **Amphojel** | Wyeth-Ayerst Laboratories, USA | aluminum hydroxide | Each 5 ml tsp. contains 320 mg of aluminum hydroxide. | Shake well. Take 25 ml doses 5-6 times a day between meals and at bedtime followed by a sip of water if desired or as directed by a doctor. | Constipation, nausea, vomiting | Do not take more than the recommended dosage in 24 hours. Do not use maximum dosage of thes product for more than 2 weeks except under the advice and supervision of a doctor. |

## Antacids That Contain Calcium Carbonate

| Brand Name | Manufacturer | Generic Name | Active Ingredient(s) | Recommended Dosage | Possible Side Effects | Warning |
|---|---|---|---|---|---|---|
| **Amitone** | Lee Pharmaceuticals | calcium carbonate | Each tablet contains 420 mg of calcium carbonate. | Chew 1-2 tablets as symptoms occur or as directed by a physician. Children under 6 should consult a doctor. | Constipation, diarrhea | Do not take more than 18 tablets in a 24-hour period or use the maximum dosage for more than 2 weeks, except under the advice and supervision of a doctor. |
| **Chooz Antacid Calcium Supplement Gum Tablets** | Schering Plough Healthcare Products, Inc. | calcium carbonate | Each tablet contains 500 mg of calcium carbonate. | Adults and children 12 years of age and older chew 1-2 tablets every 2 to 4 hours, or as directed by a doctor. | Constipation, diarrhea | Do not take more than 14 tablets in a 24 hour period. Do not use the maximum dosage for more than 2 weeks except under the supervision of a doctor. |

*Antacids That Contain Calcium Carbonate (cont'd)*

| Brand Name | Manufacturer | Generic Name | Active Ingredient(s) | Recommended Dosage | Possible Side Effects | Warning |
|---|---|---|---|---|---|---|
| **Maalox Quick Dissolve Chewable Antacid Tablets** (lemon, wild berry, and assorted berry flavors) | Novartis | calcium carbonate | Each tablet contains 600 mg of calcium carbonate. | Chew 1-2 tablets as symptoms occur or as directed by a doctor. | Constipation, diarrhea | Do not take more than 12 tablets in a 24-hour period or use the maximum dosage for more than 2 weeks except under the advice and supervision of a physician. Stop use and ask a doctor if symptoms last for more than 2 weeks. |
| **Maalox Soft Chews** (cherry and chocolate flavors) | Novartis Consumer Health, Inc. | calcium carbonate | Each chew contains calcium carbonate, several flavors, preservatives, and sweeteners. | Take 1-2 chews up to 7 times per day. | Constipation, diarrhea | Statements about this product have not been evaluated by the Food and Drug Administration. This product is not intended to diagnose, treat, cure or prevent any disease. Do not use for relief of heartburn for more than 2 weeks. |

*Antacids That Contain Calcium Carbonate (cont'd)*

| Brand Name | Manufacturer | Generic Name | Active Ingredient(s) | Recommended Dosage | Possible Side Effects | Warning |
|---|---|---|---|---|---|---|
| **Children's Mylanta Upset Stomach Relief Tablets, Bubblegum flavor** | Johnson & Johnson-Merck | calcium carbonate | Each tablet cotains 400 mg calcium carbonate. | Do not use more than 3 times a day. Children 48-95 lbs or 6-11 years of age, 2 tablets. Children 24-47 lbs or 2-5 years of age, 1 tablet. Children under 24 lbs or 2 years of age, consult a doctor. | Constipation, diarrhea | Do not take more than 6 tablets (6-11 years of age), 3 tablets (2-5 years of age) in a 24-hour period or use the maximum dosage fro more than 2 weeks except under the supervision of a doctor. Do not use if you have a kidney disease except under the advice and supervision of a doctor. |
| **Surpass Antacid Chewing Gum** | Wrigley Healthcare | calcium carbonate | Each piece contains 300 mg of calcium carbonate. | Chew 1-2 pieces as symptoms occur. Repeat hourly if symptoms return or as directed by your doctor. | Constipation, diarrhea | Do not take more than 26 pieces in 24 hours or use the maximum dosage for more than 2 weeks. |

*Antacids That Contain Calcium Carbonate (cont'd)*

| Brand Name | Manufacturer | Generic Name | Active Ingredient(s) | Recommended Dosage | Possible Side Effects | Warning |
|---|---|---|---|---|---|---|
| **Titralac Extra Strength Antacid Tablets** | 3M Healthcare | calcium carbonate | Each tablet contains 750 mg of calcium carbonate. | Take 1 or 2 tablets every 2-3 hours as symptoms occur or as directed by a doctor. Tablets can be chewed, swallowed or allowed to melt in the mouth. | Constipation, diarrhea | Do not take more than 10 tablets in a 24-hour period or use maximum dosage for more than 2 weeks, except under the advice and supervision of a doctor. |
| **Titralac Instant Relief Antacid Tablets** | 3M Healthcare | calcium carbonate | Each tablet contains 420 mg of calcium carbonate. | Take 2 tablets every 2-3 hours as symptoms occur or as directed by a doctor. Can be chewed, swallowed or allowed to melt in the mouth. | Constipation, diarrhea | Do not take more than 19 tablets in a 24-hour period or use maximum dosage for more than 2 weeks, except under supervision of a doctor. |

Antacids *That Contain Calcium Carbonate (cont'd)*

| Brand Name | Manufacturer | Generic Name | Active Ingredient(s) | Recommended Dosage | Possible Side Effects | Warning |
|---|---|---|---|---|---|---|
| **Titralac Plus, Antacid & Anti-Gas Relief Tablets** | 3M Healthcare | calcium carbonate | Each tablet conatains 400 mg of calcium carbonate, 21 mg of simethicone, and 168 mg of elemental calcium. | 2 tablets every 2 or 3 hours as symptoms occur or as directed by a doctor. Tablets can be chewed, swallowed or allowed to melt in the mouth. | Constipation, diarrhea | Do not take more than 19 tablets in a 24-hour period or use maximum dosage for more than 2 weeks except under the advice and supervision of a doctor. |
| **Tums Antacid/ Calcium Supplement** | GlaxoSmithKline | calcium carbonate | Each tablet contains 500 mg of calcium carbonate and 200 mg of elemental calcium. | Chew 2-4 tablets as symptoms occur. Repeat hourly if symptoms return, or as directed by a doctor. | Constipation, diarrhea | Do not take more than 15 tablets in a 24-hour period or use the maximum dosage of this product for more than 2 weeks except under the advice and supervision of a doctor. If symptoms persist for 2 weeks, stop using this product and see a doctor. |

## Antacids That Contain Calcium Carbonate (cont'd)

| Brand Name | Manufacturer | Generic Name | Active Ingredient(s) | Recommended Dosage | Possible Side Effects | Warning |
|---|---|---|---|---|---|---|
| **Tums E-X Extra Strength Antacid/Calcium Supplement** (orange, sugar free, and berries flavor) | GlaxoSmithKline | calcium carbonate | Each tablet contains 750 mg of calcium carbonate and 300 mg of elemental calcium. | Chew 2-4 tablets as symptoms occur. Repeat hourly if symptoms return, or as directed by a doctor. | Constipation, diarrhea | Do not take more than 9 tablets in a 24-hour period or use the maximum dosage for more than 2 weeks except under the advice and supervision of a doctor. If symptoms persist for 2 weeks, stop using the product and see a doctor. |

## Antacids That Contain Magnesium Hydroxide

| Brand Name | Manufacturer | Generic Name | Active Ingredient(s) | Recommended Dosage | Possible Side Effects | Warning |
|---|---|---|---|---|---|---|
| **Ex-Lax Milk of Magnesia Laxative/ Antacid** (chocolate crème and mint flavor) | Novartis Consumer Health, Inc. | magnesium hydroxide | Each tsp. contains 400 mg of magnesium hydroxide and 1 mg of sodium. | Adults over age 12, 1-3 tsps. up to 4 times daily. | Nausea, diarrhea | Do not take more than 12 tsps. in 24 hours or use the maximum dosage for more than 2 weeks. Ask a doctor before use if you have kidney disease. Stop use and ask a doctor if symptoms last for more than 2 weeks. |

## Antacids That Contain Magnesium Hydroxide (cont'd)

| Brand Name | Manufacturer | Generic Name | Active Ingredient(s) | Recommended Dosage | Possible Side Effects | Warning |
|---|---|---|---|---|---|---|
| **Phillips Milk of Magnesia Tablets** | Bayer Corporation | magnesium hydroxide | Each tablet contains 311 mg of magnesium hydroxide. | Chew or suck 2-4 tablets, repeat as necessary. Maximum dosage is 16 tablets in 24 hours (for children 6-12, maximum dosage is no more than 8 tablets in 24 hours. Not recommended for children under 6. | Nausea, diarrhea | Do not take more than the maximum recommended daily dosage in a 24 hour period or use the maximum dosage for more than 2 weeks. Do not use if you have kidney disease except under the advice and supervision of a doctor. |
| **Phillips Milk of Magnesia Liquid** (vanilla and original flavors) | Bayer Corporation | magnesium hydroxide | Each tsp. contains 400 mg of magnesium hydroxide. | Adults/Children 12 years and older, 1-3 tsps. with a little water up to 4 times a day or as directed by a doctor. | Nausea, diarrhea | Same as for Phillips tablets above. |

*Antacids That Contain Calcium Carbonate and Magnesium Hydroxide*

| Brand Name | Manufacturer | Generic Name | Active Ingredient(s) | Recommended Dosage | Possible Side Effects | Warning |
|---|---|---|---|---|---|---|
| **Di-Gel Antacid and Anti-gas, Tablets** (lemon orange flavor) | Schering-Plough HealthCare Products | calcium carbonate, magnesium hydroxide | Each tablet contains 280 mg of calcium carbonate, 128 mg of magnesium hydroxide, and 20 mg of simethicone. | Chew 2-4 tablets every 2 hours, after or between meals and at bedtime, or as directed by a doctor. | Diarrhea or constipation | Do not take more than 24 tablets in a 24 hour period or use the maximum dosage for more than 2 weeks or use if you have kidney disease, except under the advice and supervision of a doctor. |
| **Mylanta Antacid Gelcaps** | Johnson & Johnson-Merck | calcium carbonate, magnesium hydroxide | Each gelcap contains 550 mg of calcium carbonate, and 125 mg of magnesium hydroxide. | Swallow 2-4 gelcaps as needed or as directed by a doctor. | Diarrhea or constipation | Do not take more than 12 gelcaps in a 24-hour period or use the maximum dosage for more than 2 weeks. Do not use this product if you have kidney disease, except under the advice and supervision of a doctor. |

*Antacids that contain Calcium Carbonate and Magnesium Hydroxide (cont'd)*

| Brand Name | Manufacturer | Generic Name | Active Ingredient(s) | Recommended Dosage | Possible Side Effects | Warning |
|---|---|---|---|---|---|---|
| **Mylanta Maximum Strength Antacid Tablets** (cherry crème and cool mint flavors) | Johnson & Johnson-Merck | calcium carbonate, magnesium hydroxide | Each tablet contains 700 mg of calcium carbonate and 300 mg of magnesium hydroxide. | Thoroughly chew 2-4 tablets between meals, at bedtime or as directed by a doctor. | Diarrhea or constipation | Do not take more than 10 tablets in a 24-hour period or use the maximum dosage for more than two weeks. Do not use this product if you have kidney disease, except under the advise and supervision of a doctor. |
| **Mylanta Supreme Antacid** (cherry flavor) | Johnson & Johnson-Merck | calcium carbonate, magnesium hydroxide | Each tsp. contains 400 mg of calcium carbonate and 135 mg of magnesium hydroxide. | Shake well. Take 2-4 tsps. between meals, at bedtime or as directed by a doctor. | Diarrhea or constipation | Do not take more than 18 teaspoonfuls in a 24-hour period or use the maximum dosage for more than 2 weeks. Do not use this product except under the advice and supervision of a doctor if you have kidney disease. |

*Antacids that contain Calcium Carbonate and Magnesium Hydroxide (cont'd)*

| Brand Name | Manufacturer | Generic Name | Active Ingredient(s) | Recommended Dosage | Possible Side Effects | Warning |
|---|---|---|---|---|---|---|
| **Rolaids Antacid Tablets,** (cherry, original peppermint, and spearmint flavors) | Pfizer | calcium carbonate, magnesium hydroxide | Each tablet contains 550 mg of calcium carbonate and 110 mg of magnesium hydroxide. | Chew 1-4 tablets as symptoms occur. Repeat hourly if symptoms return, or as directed by a doctor. | Diarrhea or constipation | Do not take more than 12 tablets in a 24-hour period or use the maximum dosage for more than 2 weeks except under the advice and supervision of a doctor. |
| **Rolaids Extra Strength Antacid Tablets** (tropical punch, cool strawberry, fresh mint, and fruit flavors) | Pfizer | calcium carbonate, magnesium hydroxide | Each tablet contains 675 mg of calcium carbonate and 135 mg of magnesium hydroxide. | Chew 2-4 tablets, hourly, as needed. | Diarrhea or constipation | Do not take more than 10 tablets in a 24-hour period or use the maximum dosage for more than 2 weeks, except under the advice and supervision of a doctor. |

*Antacids That Contain Aluminum and Magnesium*

| Brand Name | Manufacturer | Generic Name | Active Ingredient(s) | Recommended Dosage | Possible Side Effects | Warning |
|---|---|---|---|---|---|---|
| **Gaviscon Regular Strength Antacid Tablets** | GlaxoSmithKline | aluminum hydroxide, magnesium trisilicate | Each tablet contains 80 mg of aluminum hydroxide and 20 mg of magnesium trisilicate. Also contains approximately 0.9 mEq sodium. | Chew 2-4 tablets 4 times a day or as directed by a doctor. Tablets should be taken after meals and at bedtime or as needed. For best results follow by a half glass of water or other liquid. Do not swallow whole. | Constipation or diarrhea | Do not take more than 16 tablets in a 24-hour period or 16 tablets daily for more than 2 weeks or if you are on a sodium-restricted diet except under the advice and supervision of a doctor. |
| **Gaviscon Extra Strength Antacid** (cool mint flavor liquid) | GlaxoSmithKline | aluminum hydroxide, magnesium carbonate | Each 2 tsps. contain 508 mg of aluminum hydroxide and 547 mg of magnesium carbontae. Also contains approximately 0.8 mEq sodium. | Shake well before using. Take 2-4 tsps. 4 times a day or as directed by a doctor. Should be taken after meals and at bedtime followed by half a glass of water. Dispense only by spoon or other measuring device. | Constipation or diarrhea | Do not take more than 16 teaspoonfuls in a 24-hour period or 16 teaspoonfuls daily for more than 2 weeks, or if you are on a sodium-restricted diet, except under the advice and supervision of a doctor. |

*Antacids That Contain Aluminum and Magnesium (cont'd)*

| Brand Name | Manufacturer | Generic Name | Active Ingredient(s) | Recommended Dosage | Possible Side Effects | Warning |
|---|---|---|---|---|---|---|
| **Gelusil Antacid, Anti-gas Tablets** | Pfizer | aluminum hydroxide, magnesium hydroxide, simethicone | Each tablet contains 200 mg of aluminum hydroxide, 200 mg of magnesium hydroxide, and 20 mg of simethicone. | Chew 2-4 tablets 1 hour after meals and at bedtime or as directed by a doctor. | Constipation or diarrhea | Do not take more than 12 tablets in a 24-hour period or use the maximum dosage for more than 2 weeks or if you have kidney disease, except under the advice and supervision of a doctor. |
| **Maalox Liquid Regular Strength Antacid/ Antigas** (cooling mint flavor) | Novartis Consumer Health, Inc. | aluminum hydroxide, magnesium hydroxide, simethicone | Each tsp. contains 200 mg of aluminum hydroxide, 200 mg of magnesium hydroxide, and 20 mg of simethicone. | Shake well. Adults 12 and older, take 2-4 tsps 4 times a day or as directed by a doctor. | Constipation or diarrhea | Do not take more than 16 teaspoonsful in 24 hours or the maximum dosage for more than 2 weeks. Children under 12, consult a doctor. Stop using if symptoms last for more than 2 weeks. Ask a doctor before use if you have kidney disease. |

*Antacids That Contain Aluminum and Magnesium (cont'd)*

| Brand Name | Manufacturer | Generic Name | Active Ingredient(s) | Recommended Dosage | Possible Side Effects | Warning |
|---|---|---|---|---|---|---|
| **Maalox Max Liquid Maximum Strength Antacid plus Antigas** (Cherry, peaches and cream, vanilla cream, and wild berry flavor) | Novartis Consumer Health, Inc. | aluminum hydroxide, magnesium hydroxide, simethicone | Each tsp. contains 400 mg of aluminum hydroxide, 400 mg of magnesium hydroxide, and 40 mg of simethicone. | Shake well. Adults over 12 years, take 2-4 tsps. 4 times a day or as directed by a doctor. | Constipation or diarrhea | Do not take more than 12 tsps. in 24 hours or use the maximum dosage for more than 2 weeks. Children under 12 consult a doctor. Stop use and ask a doctor if symptoms last for more than 2 weeks. Ask a doctor before use if you have kidney disease. |
| **Mylanta Antacid Anti-Gas Liquid** (cherry and cool mint flavors) | Johnson & Johnson-Merck | aluminum hydroxide, magnesium hydroxide, simethicone | Each 5 ml tsp. contains 200 mg of aluminum hydroxide, 200 mg of magnesium hydroxide, and 20 mg of simethicone. | Shake well. Take 2-4 tsps. between meals, at bedtime or as directed by a doctor. | Constipation or diarrhea | Do not take more than 24 tsps. in a 24-hour period or use the maximum dosage for more than 2 weeks. |

*Antacids That Contain Aluminum and Magnesium (cont'd)*

| Brand Name | Manufacturer | Generic Name | Active Ingredient(s) | Recommended Dosage | Possible Side Effects | Warning |
|---|---|---|---|---|---|---|
| **Mylanta Extra Strength Antacid Anti-Gas Liquid, Original** | Johnson & Johnson-Merck | aluminum hydroxide, magnesium hydroxide, simethicone | Each tsp. contains 400 mg of aluminum hydroxide, 400 mg of magnesium hydroxide, and 40 mg of simethicone. | Shake well. Take 2-4 tsps. between meals and at bedtime or as directed by a doctor. | Constipation or diarrhea | Do not use more than 12 tsps. in a 24-hour period or use the maximum dose of this product for more than 2 weeks or if you have kidney disease, consult your doctor. |
| **Riopan Plus Antiacid and Gas Relief Liquid** | Wyeth Ayerst Laboratories | magaldrate, simethicone | Each tsp. contains 540 mg of magaldrate and 40 mg of simethicone. | Take 1-2 tsps. between meals and at bedtime or as directed by a doctor. | Chalky taste | Dispense by spoon only. Do not ingest directly from the bottle. Do not take more than 12 tsps. in a 24-hour period or use the maximum dosage for more than 2 weeks or if you have kidney disease except under the advice and supervision of a doctor. |

## Antacids That Contain Aluminum and Magnesium (cont'd)

| Brand Name | Manufacturer | Generic Name | Active Ingredient(s) | Recommended Dosage | Possible Side Effects | Warning |
|---|---|---|---|---|---|---|
| Riopan Plus Double Strength Antacid and Antigas Relief Liquid | Wyeth Ayerst Laboratories | magaldrate, simethicone, potassium citrate | Each tsp. contains 1080 mg of magaldrate, 40 mg of simethicone and potassium cit- | Take 1 or 2 tsps. between meals and at bedtime or as directed by a doctor. | Constipation or diarrhea | Warnings same as those for Riopan Plus Antacid and Antigas Relief above. |

## Antacids That Contain Bismuth

Products that are frequently taken for diarrhea can also prove an effective treatment for acid reflux.

| Brand Name | Manufacturer | Generic Name | Active Ingredient(s) | Recommended Dosage | Possible Side Effects | Warning |
|---|---|---|---|---|---|---|
| Pepto-Bismol, Regular Strength Liquid | Proctor & Gamble | bismuth subsalicylate | Each tsp. contains 262 mg of bismuth and 130 mg of subsalicylate. | Adults 2 tbls., Children 9-12 years, 1 tbl., 6-9 years 2 tsps., 3-6 years 1 tsp. Under 3 years, ask a doctor. Repeat above dosage every hour as needed to a maximum of 8 doses in a 24-hour period. Drink plenty of clear fluids. | Black stools, darkening of the tongue | Children and teenagers who have or are recovering from chicken pox or flu should not use this medicine to treat nausea or vomiting. If nausea or vomiting is present, consult a doctor as this could be an early sign of Reye Syndrome, a rare, but serious, illness. Contains salicylates. If taken with aspirin and ringing in the ears occurs, stop using. |

## Antacids That Contain Bismuth (cont'd)

Products that are frequently taken for diarrhea can also prove an effective treatment for acid reflux.

| Brand Name | Manufacturer | Generic Name | Active Ingredient(s) | Recommended Dosage | Possible Side Effects | Warning |
|---|---|---|---|---|---|---|
| **Pepto-Bismol, Maximum Strength Liquid** | Proctor & Gamble | bismuth subsalicylate | Each tbl. contains 525 mg of bismuth subsalicylate and 236 mg of salicylate. | Shake well before using. Adults 2 tbls. Children 9-12 years of age 1 tbl, 6-9 years 2 tsps., 3-6 years 1 tsp., under 3 years ask a doctor. | Dark stools, darkening of the tongue | Children and teenagers who have or are recovering from chicken pox or flu should not use this medicine to treat nausea or vomiting. If nausea or vomiting is present, consult a doctor as it could be an early sign of Reye Syndrome, a rare, but serious, illness. This product contains salicylates. If taken with aspirin and ringing in the ears occurs, stop using. |
| **Pepto-Bismol Chewable Tablets** (cherry flavor) | Proctor & Gamble | bismuth subsalicylate | Each tablet contains 262 mg of bismuth subsalicylate and 99 mg of salicylate. | Adults 2 tablets, Children 9-12, 1 tablet, 6-9, 2/3 tablet, 3-6, 1/3 tablet. Under 3 years of age, ask a doctor. Chew or dissolve in mouth. Repeat every 1/2 to 1 hour as needed to a maximum of 8 doses in a 24-hour period. | Dark stools, darkening of the tongue | Same as above |

*Antacids That Contain Bismuth (cont'd)*

| Brand Name | Manufacturer | Generic Name | Active Ingredient(s) | Recommended Dosage | Possible Side Effects | Warning |
|---|---|---|---|---|---|---|
| **Pepto-Bismol Caplets** (cherry flavor) | Proctor & Gamble | bismuth subsalicylate | Each caplet contains 262 mg of bismuth subsalicylate and 99 mg of salicylate. | Adults 2 tablets, Children 9-12 years, 2/3 tablet, 3-6 years 1/3 tablet, Under 3 years, ask a doctor. Swallow caplet(s) with water. Do not chew. Repeat every 1/2 to 1 hour as needed to a maximum of 8 doses in a 24-hour period. | Dark stools, darkening of the tongue | Children and teenagers who have or are recovering from chicken pox or flu should not use this medicine to treat nausea or vomiting. If nausea or vomiting is present, consult a doctor because this could be an early sign of Reye Syndrome, a rare, but serious, illness. This product contains salicylates. If taken with aspirin and ringing in the ears occurs, stop using. |

*Antacids That Contain Sodium Bicarbonate* Sodium bicarbonate is generally a fast acting antacid, but since it is rapidly absorbed in the intestines, it may not be as useful for long term use. In addition to the brand names listed below, some patients find relief from symptoms by taking household baking soda made by manufacturers such as Arm and Hammer.

| Brand Name | Manufac-turer | Generic Name | Active Ingredient(s) | Recommended Dosage | Possible Side Effects | Warning |
|---|---|---|---|---|---|---|
| Alka-Seltzer Tablets, Antacid & Pain Relief Medicine, (Cherry flavor) | Bayer Corporation | sodium bicarbonate | 1 tablet contains 325 mg of aspirin, 1700 mg of heat treated sodium bicarbonate, sodium citrate, and analgesic sodium acetylsalicylate. | Dissolve 1 tablet in 4 oz of water. | No common side effects | Take no more than 8 tablets in a 24-hour period. If over 60 years, do not take more than 4 tablets in a 24-hour period or use maximum dosage for more than 10 days. Do not take if you are allergic to aspirin or have asthma or bleeding problems. Do not take if you take a prescription for anticoagulation, diabetes, gout, or arthritis unless directed by a doctor. If you take prescription drugs, consult your doctor before taking. If symptoms persist, recur frequently, or if you're under treatment for ulcer, consult your doctor. Children and teenagers should not use this medicine for chicken pox or flu symptoms before a doctor is consulted about Reye Syndrome, a rare but serious illness. If you consume 3 or more alcoholic drinks every day, ask your doctor whether you should take aspirin since it may cause stomach bleeding. |

*Antacids That Contain Sodium Bicarbonate (cont'd)*

| Brand Name | Manufac-turer | Generic Name | Active Ingredient(s) | Recommended Dosage | Possible Side Effects | Warning |
|---|---|---|---|---|---|---|
| **Alka-Seltzer Tablets, Antacid & Pain Relief, Original** | Bayer Corporation | sodium bicarbonate | Each tablet contains 325 mg of aspirin, 1916 mg of sodium bicarbonate, and 1,000 mg of citric acid. | Adults dissolve 2 tablets in 4 oz. of water and drink every four hours. | No common side effects | Do not exceed 8 tablets in 24 hours or if over 60 years old, 4 tablets in 24 hours. Other warnings same as those for Alka-Seltzer Tablets, Antacid & Pain Relief Medicine listed above. |
| **Alka-Seltzer Antacid and Heartburn Relief,** (lemon lime flavor) | Bayer Corporation | sodium bicarbonate | Each tablet contains 325 mg of aspirin, 1700 mg of sodium bicarbonate, and 1,000 mg of citric acid. | Place 2 tablets in 4 oz. of water. Dissolve tablets completely. Adults and children over 12, 2 tablets every 4 hours as needed or as directed by a doctor. Adults 60 years and older 2 tablets every 4 hours or as directed by a doctor. Children under 12, consult a doctor. You do not have to drink any of the residue that may remain on the bottom of the glass. | No common side effects | Do not exceed 8 tablets in 24 hours (adults). Those over 60 years do not exceed 4 tablets in 24 hours. Children under 12, consult a doctor. For other warnings see listing above for other Alka-Seltzer products. |

*Antacids That Contain Sodium Bicarbonate (cont'd)*

| Brand Name | Manufacturer | Generic Name | Active Ingredient(s) | Recommended Dosage | Possible Side Effects | Warning |
|---|---|---|---|---|---|---|
| **Alka-Seltzer Tablets, Antacid Relief, Gold** | Bayer Corporation | sodium bicarbonate | Each tablet contains 958 mg of heat treate sodium bicarbonate, 832 mg of citric acid, and 312 mg of potassium bicarbonate. | Dissolve 2 tablets in 4 oz of water. Adults, 2 tablets every 4 hours as needed. Children, 1/2 tablet or as directed by a doctor. You do not have to drink any of the residue that may be on the bottom of the glass. | No common side effects | If you are taking a prescription drug, do not take this product without checking with your doctor or other health professional. See other warnings from Alka-Seltzer products above. |
| **Brioschi Effervescent Antacid** (lemon flavor) | Brioschi | sodium bicarbonate | Each capful contains 269 mg of sodium bicarbonate and 770 mg of sodium. | Place 1 or 2 heaping capfuls in 1/2 glass of cool water once each hour as directed by a doctor. Drink while effervescing. Take before retiring and/or arising. | No common side effects | Do not take more than 6 capfuls in a 24 hour period or use the maximum dosage of this product for more than 2 weeks except under the supervision of a doctor. Persons 60 years or older use 1/2 max. dosage. Only use under the supervision of a doctor if you are on a sodium restricted diet. |

*Antacids That Contain Sodium Bicarbonate (cont'd)*

| Brand Name | Manufac- turer | Generic Name | Active Ingredient(s) | Recommended Dosage | Possible Side Effects | Warning |
|---|---|---|---|---|---|---|
| **Bromo - Seltzer** | Numark Laboratories | sodium bicarbonate | Each packet con- tains 650 mg of acetaminophen, 267 mg of citric acid, and 350 mg of sodium bicar- bonate. | Adults 12 years and over pour 1 packet into an empty glass. Add half a glass of cold water. Dissolve gran- ules completely before drinking. Repeat every 4 hours as needed or as directed by a doctor. Maximum recom- mended dose is 3 packets per day (2 packets per day if you are over 60. | No common side effects | Do not take more than 3 packets per day if under 60 years old (2 packets per day if over 60) except under the supervision of a doctor. Do not use the maximum dosage for more than 10 days or if you are on a sodium restricted diet. If you consume 3 or more alco- holic drinks every day, ask your doctor whether you should take aceta- minophen or other pain relievers/fever reducers. Acetaminophen may cause liver damage. |

*Sucralfate*

| Brand Name | Manufacturer | Generic Name | Active Ingredient(s) | Recomended Dosage | Possible Side Effects | Warning |
|---|---|---|---|---|---|---|
| **Carafate** | Aventis Pharmaceuticals | sucralfate | sucralfate | 1 g 2-4 times a day (both liquid and tablets). | Constipation | Do not take this drug if you have severe kidney disease. You should also check with your doctor before you combine Carafate with any of the following: antacids, blood-thinning drugs, cimetidine, digoxin, drugs for contrlling spasms, ketoconazole, levothyroxine, phenytoin, quinidine, quinolone, ranitidine, tetracycline, theophylline. |

*Prescription H2 Blockers*

| Brand Name | Manufacturer | Generic Name | Recommended Dosage | Possible Side Effects | Warning |
|---|---|---|---|---|---|
| Axid | Wyeth Consumer Healthcare | nizatidine | 1 tablet orally twice a day for 6-8 weeks | Abdominal pain, diarrhea, dizziness, gas, headache, indigestion, inflammation of the nose, nausea, pain, sore throat, vomiting, weakness | Could mask stomach malignancy. May not be indicated if you have severe kidney disease. |
| Pepcid | Johnson & Johnson-Merck | famotidine | 20 mg or 2.5 ml (1/2 tsp.) twice a day for up to 6 weeks. For inflammation of the esophagus due to GERD, the dose is 20-40 mg or 2.5-5 ml twice a day for up to 12 weeks. For Zollinger-Ellison Syndrome, 20 mg every 6 hours. | Headache, fatigue, drowsiness, dizziness, nausea, vomiting, abdominal pain, diarrhea, constipation | Check with your doctor before taking with Itraconazole or Ketoconazole. Could mask stomach malignancy. May not be indicated if you have severe kidney disease. |

*Prescription H2 Blockers (cont'd)*

| Brand Name | Manufacturer | Generic Name | Recommended Dosage | Possible Side Effects | Warning |
|---|---|---|---|---|---|
| Tagamet | GlaxoSmithKline | cimetidine | 1,600 mg daily divided into doses of 800 mg twice a day or 400 mg 4 times a day for 12 weeks. | Headache, fatigue, drowsiness, dizziness, nausea, vomiting, abdominal pain, diarrhea | Avoid the use of alcoholic beverages. Antacids can reduce the effect of Tagamet when taken at the same time. If combined with antacids, take the antacids 2 hours before or after Tagamet. Check with your doctor before combining Tagamet with any of the following medications: antidiabetic drugs, antifungal drugs, aspirin, augmentin, tranquilizers, Beta-blocking blood pressure drugs, calcium-blocking blood pressure drugs, chlorpromazine, cisapride, cyclosporine, digoxin, medications for irregular heartbeat, metoclopramide, metronidazole, narcotic pain relievers, nicotine, paroxetine, pentoxifylline, phenytoin, quinine, sucralfate, theophylline, warfarin. |

*Prescription H2 Blockers (cont'd)*

| Brand Name | Manufac- turer | Generic Name | Recommended Dosage | Possible Side Effects | Warning |
|---|---|---|---|---|---|
| Zantac | GlaxoSmithKline | rantidine hydrochloride | 150 mg or 10 ml (2 tsps.) twice a day. For erosive esophagitis, 150 mg or 10 ml (2 tsps.) 4 times a day. For Zollinger-Ellison Syndrome, 150 mg of 10 ml (2 tsps.) twice a day. | Headache, fatigue, drowsiness, nausea, vomiting, abdominal pain, diarrhea, constipation Do not take if you have kidney or liver disease. | Check with your doctor before combining Zantac with alcohol, blood thinning drugs, diazepam, diltiazem, enoxacin, glipizide, glyburide, itraconazole, ketoconazole, metformin, nifedipine, phenytoin, procainamide, sucralfate, theophylline, triazolam. |

*Over–The–Counter H2 Blockers*

| Brand Name | Manufac- turer | Generic Name | Recommended Dosage | Possible Side Effects | Warning |
|---|---|---|---|---|---|
| Axid AR | Wyeth Consumer Healthcare | nizatidine, 75mg | Swallow 1 tablet with water 1/2-1 hour before eating food and beverages that cause you heartburn. Can be used up to twice daily (up to 2 tablets in 24 hours). | Headache, fatigue, drowsiness, dizziness, nausea, vomiting, abdominal pain, diarrhea, constipation | Do not take the maximum daily dosage for more than 2 weeks continuously unless directed by a doctor. If you are pregnant or nursing a baby, seek the advice of a health professional before using. |

*Over-The-Counter H2 Blockers (cont'd)*

| Brand Name | Manufacturer | Generic Name | Recommended Dosage | Possible Side Effects | Warning |
|---|---|---|---|---|---|
| **Pepcid AC** | Johnson & Johnson-Merck | famotidine | Swallow 1 tablet with water. Take 1 tablet 1 hour before a meal that could cause symptoms. | Headache, fatigue, drowsiness, dizziness, nausea, vomiting, abdominal pain, diarrhea, constipation | Take no more than 2 tablets per day. Do not give to children under 12. |
| **Tagamet HB** | GlaxoSmithKline | cimetidine | 2 tablets taken with water once or up to twice a day. | Headache, abdominal pain, diarrhea, constipation | Do not take more than 4 tablets in 24 hours. Do not give to children under 12 unless your doctor prescribes this medication. |
| **Zantac 75** | GlaxoSmithKline | ranitidine 75 mg | Swallow 1 tablet with water. Do not chew. Can be used up to twice daily (up to 2 tablets in 24 hours). | Headache, fatigue, drowsiness, nausea, vomiting, abdominal pain, diarrhea, constipation | Do not take the maximum daily dose for more than 14 consecutive days, unless directed by your doctor. If you have trouble swallowing or persistent abdominal pain, see your doctor promptly. |

*Prescription Proton Pump Inhibitors*

| Brand Name | Manufacturer | Generic Name | Recommended Dosage | Possible Side Effects | Warning |
|---|---|---|---|---|---|
| **Aciphex** | Janssen | rabeprazole sodium | 20 mg once a day for 4-8 weeks. | Headache, diarrhea, abdominal pain | Possible drug interaction with Cyclosporine, Ketoconazole, Digoxin. |
| **Nexium** | AstraZeneca, LP | esomeprazole magnesium | 40 mg once a day. | Headache, diarrhea, abdominal pain | Women should not take this mediation if they plan on becoming pregnant. It is unknown if this medication is excreted in breast-milk. A doctor should be consulted about possible risks to the fetus. |
| **Prevacid** | TAP Pharmaceuticals | lansoprazole | 15-30 mg once a day for up to 8 weeks. For erosive esophagitis, take 30 mg daily, before eating for up to 8 weeks. For Zollinger-Ellison Syndrome, take 60 mg once a day. | Headache, Diarrhea, abdominal pain | Check with your doctor before combining Prevacid with Ampicillin, Digoxin, Iron salts, Ketoconazole, sucralfate or theophylline. |
| **Prilosec** | AstraZeneca | omeprazole | 20 mg once a day. | Abdominal pain, diarrhea, headache, nausea, vomiting | Long term use can cause severe stomach inflammation. Check with your doctor before combining Prilosec with Ampicillin-containing drugs, cyclosporine, diazepam, disulfiram, iron, ketoconazole, phynytoin, coumadin. |

## Prescription Proton Pump Inhibitors (cont'd)

| Brand Name | Manufacturer | Generic Name | Recommended Dosage | Possible Side Effects | Warning |
|---|---|---|---|---|---|
| **Protonix** | Wyeth-Ayerst Pharmaceuticals | pantoprazole | 40 mg orally once a day | Headache, diarrhea, abdominal pain | May interfere with the absorption of drugs such as ketoconazole, ampicillin and iron salts. |

## Over-The-Counter Proton Pump Inhibitors

| Brand Name | Manufacturer | Generic Name | Recommended Dosage | Possible Side Effects | Warning |
|---|---|---|---|---|---|
| **Prilosec** | Kremers Urban Development Co. | omeprazole | 10 mg, 20 mg, or 40 mg delayed realease capsules. | Abdominal pain, diarrhea, headache, nausea, vomiting | Long term use can cause severe stomach inflammation. Check with your doctor before combining Prilosec with Ampicillin-containing drugs, cyclosporine, diazepam, disulfiram, iron, ketoconazole, phynytoin, coumadin. |

# 11

# UNDERSTANDING YOUR MEDICATION
## *The Basics*

B OTH OVER-THE-COUNTER (OTC) AND PRE-scription medications are available for the treatment of GERD. Whichever kind you use, it's a good idea to learn about its primary ingredients as well as how and when to take it.

### *Learning More about Your Medication*

Your doctor or pharmacist is the first place you should turn with any questions about medication you take. Drug manufacturer Web sites are also good sources of information. Those sites often provide links to the same information included in package inserts; however, much of the information is written in highly technical language that may be difficult for the average person to understand. So, if you have any question about what may be contained in a particular medication or what common side effects may be, contact your pharmacist or doctor.

You can also find information about GERD medications on Web sites maintained by individuals. Although much of the information may be correct, some of it may be based more on the personal opinion of the site's host than on scientific research. Your prescribing physician and pharmacist are better sources of information for your drug related questions. Web sites we recommended without hesitation are those of the American Gastroenterological Association (http://www.gastro.org), the American College of Gastroenterology (www.acg.gi.org), and the American Medical Association (www.ama-assn.org).

## Determining What's in a Medication

The labels of non-prescription drugs are required by law to list all of the ingredients in the medication. Before taking any medication, read the label carefully because it may warn about chemicals or drugs in the medication that can cause allergic reactions.

Prescription medication labels do not always list all of the ingredients, but they always include both the brand name and the generic name. For example, Prilosec is a brand name. Its generic name is Omeprazole.

The labels of both prescription and non-prescription medications will also contain the name of the company that manufactures the product.

WHAT FORM OF MEDICATION SHOULD YOU TAKE?  Unlike medications for other diseases and conditions, medications for GERD are available in a wide variety of forms. Many non-prescription GERD medications are available as capsules, tablets, chewable tablets, liquids or powders that can be mixed with liquids, and even chewing gum. The disadvantage of forms of delivery such as liquids, powders, and chewable tablets is that it's sometimes difficult to be sure of the exact dosage you are getting. It is also often unclear whether taking "too much" of an over-the-counter medicine is appropriate. Therefore, it is important that you always read the labels of OTC drugs.

Most prescription medications are in capsules or tablet form. Tablets and capsules generally contain identical amounts of medication; the difference is that a capsule is a tablet that has been coated with gelatin to make it easier to swallow. Tablets and capsules have the advantage of ensuring a consistent dosage of medication. They also offer choice to patients who have a preference. The disadvantage of capsules and tablets is that some people, particularly those with diseases of the esophagus, find them difficult to swallow. Fortunately for those patients, a liquid form of just about every class of antacid does exist.

Some patients, usually those who are hospitalized, aren't able to take oral medication. In those cases, intravenous (IV) formulations—usually H2 blockers or Proton Pump Inhibitors—are available.

HOW MUCH SHOULD YOU TAKE?   By law, all medication labels, whether for prescription or OTC drugs, must include information about how much medication you should take at one time. If the medicine is a prescription, dosing and interval of dosing must also be clearly labeled. If the physician makes an error in dosing, the pharmacist usually will not dispense the drug without first confirming dosage information with the physician.

Since non-prescription medications are not intended for a specific individual, labels on those products quantify dosing amounts for both children and adults Since most dosages of medication are related to the weight of the individual, very small adults (or very large children) should probably consult their doctor about what dosage would be the most appropriate for them. In patients with kidney or liver disease, dose adjustments are typically determined by the physician and/or pharmacist.

Prescriptions are written for specific individuals, and so there is usually only one dose prescribed and labeled on the bottle. Typically, the information on the bottle will read something like "Take one tablet by mouth every day." Prescription medication labels will also indicate the strength of each dose in milligrams (mg). For example, a label might read "20 mg tablets."

It is very important that you pay attention to the dosages specified on the label of your medications. The dosage on the label of a prescription bottle is not a suggested dosage, it is the exact dosage your doctor wants you to take. Do not take more or less than the prescribed dosage without first consulting your prescribing physician. Even if you feel that the medication is not working as well as you had hoped, do not change the dosage without consulting your doctor.

As we noted above, non-prescription medications are not designed for any particular individual; however, they still make specific recommendations about dosages and you should pay attention to what they say. Typically, they will indicate a maximum amount. For example, the label might say "Repeat every half hour to a maximum of eight dosages in 24 hours." You should not exceed this maximum. If the medication is not working, call your doctor. Also, watch out for side effects listed on the warning label of the medication.

WHEN SHOULD YOU TAKE YOUR MEDICATION?   Whether you are taking a prescription or a non-prescription medicine, the label will tell you when you should take it. The most common recommendations are:

That the medication be taken at a specific time, for example "one tablet in the morning and one tablet at night."

That the medication be taken prior to or after a specific event, for example, "one tablet one half hour before a meal."

That the medication be taken when experiencing symptoms, for example, "take one tablet if you experience stomach upset."

HOW SHOULD YOU STORE YOUR MEDICATION?   In most cases, medications may be stored in your purse or briefcase or on the shelf of your medicine cabinet. Some medications need to be refrigerated. If that is the case, that information will be printed on the label. Be sure to store your medications properly. Failure to do so may cause them to lose their effectiveness.

**Do GERD Medications React Adversely with Other Drugs or Food?**   Many medications either lose effectiveness or cause unpleasant side effects if they are taken in combination with other drugs or some foods. This information will appear on the labels of both prescription and non-prescription medications. Such a warning might read, "Do not take this medication in combination with alcohol." As a general rule, alcohol, illicit drugs, or accompanying co-administered medicines can all interact with the drug and impact its effectiveness. Coexisting intake of such substances may also increase or decrease the therapeutic levels of the drug causing increased side effects or may reduce the intended effect of the drug.

**Who Should Not Take a Medication?**   If a doctor has prescribed a medication, he or she has determined that it is appropriate for you. Through your face-to-face consultation and by studying your medical history, your doctor will know what medications you should generally avoid. But since non-prescription medications are intended for the general public, labels on these medications will always specify not only who should take them but also who should not take them. For example, the label on a medication may read, "This medication should not be taken by women who are nursing or by people with high blood pressure."

**What Side Effects Might I Expect?**   Companies that manufacture prescription and non-prescription medications routinely include on their labels (or on an insert with a prescription) just about everything that could conceivably result from taking their products. Generally, there are so many warnings that you will probably need a magnifying glass to read all the fine print. However, it is highly unlikely that most of these things will ever happen to anyone, so you should not be unduly alarmed by the long list of warnings some medication labels include. If a side effect is common (or likely) it will appear in bold type or on a brightly colored sticker on the bottle. For example, a bottle might say, "This medication may cause drowsiness."

CAN I SHARE MY MEDICATION? Since GERD is such a common problem, many families are tempted to share the medications that work for them. If the medication is a non-prescription one, sharing may be appropriate, as long as both parties have read and understand the label, including what the correct dose is, when the medication should be taken, and what, if any, restrictions exist.

Under no circumstances should you share prescription medication with anyone. Prescription medication has been prescribed only for you. The chances are that it will not produce the desired effect for another person. There is an even greater chance that the medication could cause them harm. Please also note that it is a crime to sell your medications to someone else.

HOW LONG SHOULD I TAKE MY MEDICATION? Fortunately, antacids are among the safest medications available today. People who experience only occasional episodes of GERD may find relief from the same non-prescription medication for many years. Those who suffer frequent or intense episodes of GERD, however, should certainly see a doctor and should probably consider prescription medications. Because prescription medications are usually stronger and designed to work over a longer period of time than non-prescription drugs, they are prescribed only for a specific time (e.g. for six months). After that time is up, your pharmacy will not refill your prescription without your doctor's orders. If the medication is working well for you, your doctor can usually refill your prescription by phone. If your doctor feels that you should have an examination before you continue taking any more of the medication, he or she will not refill your prescription without an office visit.

Physicians have a responsibility to see and examine their patients in the office setting at least every six to 12 months, particularly if symptoms are persistent, and to review the history and response to drug and lifestyle changes previously discussed. Many physicians will not as a rule prescribe medicines for longer than six to 12 months without an office evaluation.

The label on your prescription bottle will tell you how often your prescription can be refilled.

**WHAT IF I EXPERIENCE SIDE EFFECTS?**  Generally speaking, if you begin to experience side effects, stop taking the medication and contact your doctor immediately. If you experience severe side effects and cannot reach your doctor, get to a hospital emergency room.

**DO MEDICATIONS EXPIRE?**  Although most medications today last a long time, they can, and do, lose their effectiveness over time. The law requires that all medications, prescription or non-prescription, include an expiration date on the label of the bottle.

If your medication has passed that date, ask your doctor for a new prescription. Throw away any medication whose expiration date has passed.

**ARE PRESCRIPTION MEDICATIONS ALWAYS MORE EFFECTIVE THAN OTC MEDICATIONS?**  Non-prescription or OTC medications are designed for the general public, not for a specific individual. Because most people experience GERD on an occasional and mild basis, they only need a product that will work for a short period of time (30 minutes or so) But that's enough for most people.

Prescription medications, on the other hand, are intended to be prescribed on an individual basis to patients that experience frequent, prolonged or very severe episodes of GERD. For these patients the problem is seldom just an extra spicy dinner. Sometimes the real problem is that the antacids they've been taking for a long time have concealed a more serious problem. Whatever the cause, these people will require a prescription medication that will need to be taken with greater regularity than non-prescription medications.

Many drugs that were formerly only available by prescription are now available over-the-counter. That OTC version of such a drug, however, is generally not as strong as the prescription product.

Be careful not to "self-treat" your symptoms with over the counter doses greater than those recommended on the bottle. If you find that symptomatic relief can only be attained with doses above that recommended as a maximal dose on the bottle, you should seek assistance from you physician.

IS ONE MEDICATION ENOUGH TO TREAT MY GERD?  Generally, people with mild or occasional episodes of GERD find relief from a single non-prescription product. And, in fact, it is generally recommended that a GERD sufferer stick to a single product, since taking several products simultaneously can often cause adverse reactions or make the problem worse.

For people who experience severe or frequent GERD, however, a combination of medications may be appropriate. For example, some patients may require proton pump inhibitors twice a day, with an additional dose of an H2 blocker at bedtime, a regimen that has been shown to adequately suppress acid in those with severe GERD. Others may require both a proton pump inhibitor (or H2 blocker) and a pro-motility agent for maximal acid suppression. Such combinations of medications are only given, however, if the doctor has carefully examined the patient and continues to closely monitor the patient's progress.

# 12

# COMPLEMENTARY &
# ALTERNATIVE MEDICINE
## *Non-Traditional Choices*

FOR MANY YEARS, "ALTERNATIVE" MEDICINE was anything mainstream doctors didn't understand or approve of. Today, many doctors are beginning to view some forms of alternative medicine to be, as its name suggests, another choice. Within the last 10 years or so, some mainstream doctors, hospitals, and clinics have even begun to include therapies such as acupuncture, chiropractic, therapeutic massage, and various kinds of relaxation techniques within their range of services.

Because these treatments are generally prescribed in addition to a traditional course of treatment, these therapies are usually referred to as "complementary" rather than alternative medicines.

### The Origins of Alternative Medicine

Throughout most of human history (and to some extent, even today) finding anything that was effective in treating a disease or condition was a matter of trial and error. The remedies that didn't work were probably buried along with the unfortunate patient, while the remedies that achieved the desired result were passed along to future generations. Those who had the best record at providing cures and treatments on a more   predictable basis formed the foundation of the science of medicine. Those who practiced the healing arts also soon began to mix the herbs and other substances that had proven effective in prior generations to achieve a yet better outcome. They became, in effect, the world's first pharmacists.

## Prescientific Theories of Medicine

Since healing was often considered a miracle—in part magic—many cultures considered healers and healing to have a spiritual and religious component. So early on, the practice of medicine took on a spiritual point of view as potions, powders, and even prayers were thought to be effective in healing ailments.

Early philosophical works based on the understanding of the human body also led to a belief that the body contained some sort of inner energy. All bodily functions were assumed to be affected positively or negatively by the natural elements that people could experience first hand, such as air, water, earth and fire.

The Greek philosopher Hippocrates believed that the body was made up of four "humors"—blood, phlegm, yellow bile, and black bile—and that an imbalance of those humors was the basis for disease. Others at that time, however, thought that disease was "sent by the gods" and, thus, that all cures could only be determined by them. When the Romans conquered the Greeks, the Romans adopted those ideas, too. They also began to experiment with herbs and other remedies, and even came to understand that cleanliness (the avoidance of dirt) led to a healthier life. Out of this belief system came the notion of "civilized society" that included the creation of baths, aqueducts, and sophisticated sewer systems.

To these basic beliefs were added further philosophical interpretations of what forces were responsible for life and bodily function.

Galen, a philosopher and physician born in 129 AD, became the unchallenged authority on medicine for the next thousand years. Although not religious himself, he nonetheless regarded the body as the instrument of the soul and believed that "pneuma" (breath and air) formed the fundamental principal of life.

## The Origins of Mainstream Medicine

It was not Galen, however, who first described the circulation of blood through the body. It was the English physician, William Harvey, who discovered in the seventeenth century that the circulation of the blood throughout the body was the basic "humor" or life, or life sustaining function. From Harvey came a new understanding of both blood and circulation: the path by which disease could travel to multiple organs within the body.

Before long, his ideas developed into a formal belief system which, along with a pharmacoepia (known inventory of drugs, chemicals and treatments) shaped the mainstream practice of medicine.

Alternative medicine arose from dissatisfaction with the at-times unsuccessful efforts of the mainstream practitioners. The realization that "mainstream" medicine was not necessarily the right choice for all patients with ailments began to form a rift in what was understood as the "accepted" therapies for particular ailments. A new group of practitioners emerged to offer "alternative" therapies. These therapies were founded on the basic presumption that herbs and vitamins, along with other non-traditional healing modalities, such as Yoga and acupuncture were the basis for a newer more therapeutic source of healing.

The questions raised against traditional medicine centuries ago are still being raised today. Over time, we have begun to learn that alternatives to traditional medicine, although not a replacement for "mainstream" medicine, can clearly be helpful as an adjunctive or complementary approach to treating bodily ailments.

## Gastroenterology

Physicians are the representatives of the mainstream practice of medicine for our time. They are educated in medical schools and then serve an apprenticeship where learn to apply their education by studying with those who have had more experience. A doctor who practices in gastroenterology, for instance, must complete four years of medical school, followed by a three-year residency in internal medicine, followed by a three-year fellowship in gastroenterology. Only after passing board exams in both internal medicine and gastroenterology, can a gastroenterologist be licensed to practice.

In traditional mainstream medicine reliance is based on treatments and medicines that have stood the test of time and have been formally approved for use in our country by agencies like the Food and Drug Administration (FDA) and are recommended by organizations within our specialty.

Although modern day physicians know more about how the human body works than did any other generation of previous doctors, they still don't know everything. As hard as they try and as much as they learn, there are still some cures that remain beyond their reach.

## Incorporating Alternative Medicine into Physician Training

Until recently, there was very little interest in studying the effect of alternative medicine and its place in the treatment of patients. However, most medical schools are now training physicians to understand not only the philosophical basis of treatment and disease, but to study the effects of alternative treatments on patients with ailments. Currently, a large number of studies is emerging that specifically examine the effect alternative medicines have on patient well-being for both physical and mental health.

## "Natural" Medicines

There will always be people who are skeptical of traditional "chemical" medicines that mainstream physicians prescribe. Many people are afraid of medicines, regardless of the source, but some patients are particularly skeptical if the treatment is pharmacologically produced. To meet the demand for what they consider more "natural" treatments, some individuals and large companies have formulated medicinal agents from plants and a variety of other materials. These natural treatments, whether or not they have been scientifically tested to prove that they work, at least claim to have met the test of being produced "naturally." The problem is that in the United States and other countries some manufacturers of these alternative medicines have marketed products that have little scientific support and may, in fact, even be harmful.

Since following a doctor's recommendation is voluntary, some people will also choose not to follow a course of treatment that is recommended, despite a multitude of scientific data to support not only its benefit, but also (at times) its ability to prolong life. Instead, they will shop around for something they think will either work faster or will not require that they do what is a recommended known effective treatment, such as giving up smoking, losing weight, or taking antibiotics to treat a serious infection.

Because so many people now seek treatment from alternative medicines and practitioners of alternative therapies, traditionally trained physicians continue to study alternative therapies in large patient populations to  investigate their efficacy and safety. These studies may pave the way for more beneficial alternative therapies to become incorporated into mainstream medicine.

## Alternative/ Complementary Medicines and Therapies

Every culture has developed a slightly different approach to treating injury and illness. In North America most alternative medicines and therapies offered as part of a complementary program of care are those that originated in Asia.

CHINESE MEDICINE. Chinese medicine, which has been practiced for at least 5,000 years, is based on the belief that in all of nature there are opposing forces: night and day, hot and cold, up and down, and so on. These opposing forces are known as the Yin and Yang. Most of us are familiar with the symbol that is commonly used to illustrate this concept. The Yin is the "dark" side of nature, the Yang the "light". Like every other living thing, the human body is considered to have both Yin and Yang qualities. The liver, for example, is dark and solid and is considered a Yin organ, while the stomach, since it is hollow, is considered a Yang organ. Although it takes many years of study to fully understand the intricacies of Chinese medicine, in general it can be said that the goal of treatment is to help the patient achieve a balance between the Yin and Yang.

If you seek treatment for GERD from a practitioner of Chinese medicine, a diagnosis will be made by physical examination or possibly in the case of some practitioners by one or more of the diagnostic tests described in Chapter 5. A Chinese doctor will then probably suggest some of the lifestyle changes outlined in Chapter 14, some of the dietary changes outlined in Chapter 8 and will likely prescribe a Chinese medicine. These medicines may come in the form of herbs and plants that you will make into a tea or tablets or liquid. A Chinese doctor may also recommend that you try acupuncture.

ACUPUNCTURE. is based on the belief that every living thing contains a life force known as ch'i (pronounced chee). Ch'i flows along 14 invisible, interconnected "meridians" that exist on each side of the body and crisscross the arms, legs, trunk and head, and flow through the muscles. There are 360 points along these meridians. Where the meridians come to the surface of the skin, acupuncture points are created. Since each meridian is connected to one or more organs, stimulating one or more of the acupuncture points can positively impact that organ. Energy is constantly flowing along the meridians. A interruption or unbalance in the flow of ch'i therefore upsets the balance of the Yin and Yang and can cause discomfort or illness. Application of acupuncture restores the balance. In China, the belief in the effectiveness of acupuncture is so widespread that it is even used as an anesthetic for patients undergoing major surgery.

Although no one knows for sure exactly how acupuncture works, one theory is that application of acupuncture needles causes a release of endorphins in the brain. Endorphins are naturally produced polypeptide (protein) brain substances that can have the same effect as chemical narcotics by binding to opiate receptors thereby affecting pain. There is also some evidence that stimulating acupoints dissipates lactic acid in the muscles. In Chinese medicine, the accumulation of carbon monoxide and lactic acid in the muscles is thought to be caused by an imbalance in the influence of the five elements wood, fire, earth, water, and metal. Another theory is that acupuncture raises the levels of triglycerides, hormones, prostaglandins, white blood count and gamma globulins. Yet another theory is that acupuncture causes a release of vasodilators like histamines that dilate the blood vessels.

Whatever the actual mechanism, acupuncture is now more widely accepted than ever before as an effective alternative, or complementary, therapy. Because acupuncture needles are very thin, acupuncture is a painless procedure.

There are specific acupuncture treatments for gastrointestinal problems. These are typically on the side of the face and body. Acupuncture has reportedly been used successfully for some patients with conditions such as GERD, gastritis and nausea.

ACUPRESSURE Acupressure is based on the same principles as acupuncture. The difference is that instead of inserting needles into the acupuncture points, pressure is applied to that point for a specific period of time. One of the advantages of acupressure is that patients can be trained to do this therapy for themselves. As in acupuncture, the pressure points that affect various organs are along the meridians that exist throughout the body. For example, the pressure point for the stomach is along the left thigh.

REIKI. Reiki is another ancient healing art, originating in Japan. Those who practice Reiki, believe, as do the Chinese, that everyone's body contains a universal life energy and that problems arise when the life energy is out of balance. Reiki is somewhat like acupressure, in that practitioners of Reiki find the pressure points on the body, but instead of applying pressure, they funnel healing energy through their hands into the pressure point on the patient. This form of energy transfer is sometimes performed without even touching the recipient or Reiki patient.

AYRUVEDA. Ayruveda is a healing art that has been practiced in India for more than 5,000 years. Although it has some similarities to Chinese medicine, Ayruveda is a regimen that combines diet, herbs, cleansing and purification, Yoga, astrology and gemstones. In Chinese medicine five elements that affect health are wood, fire, earth, water and metal, in Ayruveda, elements are ether, air, fire, water and earth. These elements, combined as Vata, Pitta, and Kapha are known as the doshas or constitutional types.

Unlike Western diet plans, Ayruveda concentrates less on basic food groups and more on texture, temperature and taste, as well as paying attention to what foods are combined with others. Those who follow Ayruveda believe that overindulgence, bad combinations of food and other factors create a toxic substance known as "ama" that coats the digestive tract and tongue and causes disease.

If you consult a practitioner of Ayruveda, he or she will examine you and determine what your dosha is, then prescribe a regimen of nutrition, exercise, cleansing, preventative medicine and even clothing that will keep you healthy.

REFLEXOLOGY. Not all alternative medical systems are Eastern. Reflexology is an American healing philosophy developed by Dr. William Fitzgerald in 1917. Dr. Fitzgeralds's concept was that, as in Chinese medicine, there are certain pressure points on the body that, when massaged, can improve the function of various internal organs. Fitzgerald believed that there were ten vertical strips running the length of the body and that a problem in any one zone affected the rest of the zone. Eunice Ingham, a follower of Fitzgerald, refined this theory by concentrating on the feet. She felt that since the extremities had slower circulation, tiny crystals built up at the ends of the nerves and that crushing these crystals through massage would restore balance to the body, and thus health. Whatever justification there may be to that theory, one proven positive effect of applying pressure to various points of the feet is that the procedure is very relaxing to many people and can thus help relieve the stress that may cause an episode of GERD.

HOMEOPATHY. Homeopathy (from "homeo" meaning similar and "pathos" meaning disease) was founded by a German, Samuel Christian Hahnemann, in the late 1700s. Hahnemann's philosophy was that symptoms of a disease were signs of the body's attempt to resist disease and that the medical practitioners of his time were primarily concerned with addressing symptoms of diseases rather than the root cause of the symptoms. He called what the mainstream practitioners were doing "suppression." Hahnemann believed that the human body was usually capable of curing itself if given the right stimulation in the form of what he called "bioenergetic medicines." These medicines were minute amounts of plant, animal and mineral substances that would, in higher dosages be toxic or cause the symptoms of a disease. The idea was that once the immune system was correctly stimulated by these medicines, it would return the body to homeostasis—the same sort of balanced state achieved in Chinese medicine. Hahnemann tested his remedies on healthy people to produce symptoms, figuring that the same remedy, in a smaller dosage, would cure those same symptoms in a person who was ill.

Homeopathy takes a holistic approach to medicine, thus the homeopathic healer views the patient as a whole person taking into account everything that is going on in that person's life. Therefore, homeopathic remedies, like Chinese herbs, are prescribed on an individual basis.

Homeopathic remedies come in many forms, tablets, pellets, granules, powders, liquids, ointments, oils, gels, sprays and soaps. Since these remedies contain only minute quantities of basic ingredients, potency is measured by the amount of dilution (e.g. 2X, 10X). Homeopathic medicines are unlike "Western" medicines, in that the more diluted they are, the more potent they are.

Homeopathic medicines are considered to be especially effective for people with chronic diseases like heartburn. The basic premise of homeopathic preparations is to dilute the herb. Many of these preparations are sold in health food stores, however, no conclusive scientific data has supported their use. Because the dilution of the active herb is considered to be high, the relative risk to the consumer is considered low enough not to induce fear or anxiety if a patient seeks a homeopathic remedy for acid reflux.

Common homeopathic remedies for digestive illnesses include Ipecacuahna (made from the herb ipecac), Arsenicum (arsenic), Nux Vomica (poison nut), Podophyllum (may apple), Pulsatilla (windflower), Carbo veg (vegetable charcoal), lycopodium, Argent nit, and Natrum phos (sodium phosphate).

NATUROPATHY. As its name suggests, naturopathy is based on the theory that our bodies heal themselves the best, that is regain the inner balance that restores health, through "natural" activities like a diet of unprocessed foods, exercise, a clean environment and hydrotherapy. Naturopathic healers, unlike homeopathic healers, take advantage of Western diagnostic methods such as imaging and testing. Although some minor surgeries are considered acceptable, naturopaths do not believe in major surgery or the use of most synthetic drugs. They do recognize the value of other holistic therapies and remedies such as acupuncture, Chinese medicine and homeopathy.

Naturopaths recommend the same types of lifestyle changes as most Western physicians including eating small meals that are low in fat and avoiding foods that are known causes of heartburn. They also recommend cessation of smoking and avoidance of carbonated drinks.

Some common naturopathic remedies for GERD are: aloe vera gel and deglycherhizinated licorice (DGL).

BIOFEEDBACK. Biofeedback is a treatment in which people learn to interpret the messages their bodies are sending them and act accordingly. Originating in the 1960s, biofeedback is based on the theory that if people can learn to recognize the things that trigger symptoms of stress or the onset of a particular physiological event, that they can, by force of will, relax and prevent the event from occurring. Biofeedback is often achieved through use of a machine of some sort that measures temperature, blood pressure, perspiration, or electrical signals produced by the muscles and displays this information on a screen. The patient is taught to make internal adjustments (such as slower breathing, relaxing muscles) which bring about the desired response.

AROMATHERAPY. Because our sense of smell is such an important part of our lives, particular aromas have a strong emotional impact on most people. Although almost everything in nature has an aroma of some sort —some much stronger than others—the aromas used in aromatherapy are generally produced from pure essential oils. These are highly concentrated extracts that are either heated, burned as candles or added to hot bath water. Because aromatherapy seems to be very effective in helping some people sleep better and relax, it is now even being used to calm people with Alzheimer's Disease.

When a patient is experiencing symptoms caused by excess acidity in the digestive system, aromotherapists recommend that hot or warm compresses containing the oils of chamomile or lavender be applied to the abdomen or the oils massaged into the abdomen.

## Relaxation Therapies

YOGA. Practiced in India for thousands of years, Yoga is a relaxation technique in which, through intense concentration, the individual is able to produce and direct energy in a more positive direction. Practitioners of Yoga recommend it particularly for people with chronic diseases like GERD. The main premise of Yoga is to allow the patient to reach a point of relaxation in order to attain stress reduction, thereby assisting digestion. This approach also encourages the Yoga participant to concentrate on relaxation breathing as well as a more methodical approach to eating.

MEDITATION. Although Yoga involves meditation, those who find relaxation through meditation do not necessarily practice Yoga. While meditation is a very individual concept, in general, meditation usually involves clearing the mind of everything stressful by concentrating on breathing or visualizing pleasant things.

In the previous chapter, we discussed some of the alternative medical practices that are now being incorporated into "traditional" American medicine. Since these alternative and/or complementary therapies sometimes involve herbal medicines, in this chapter studying the more common ones will provide for a perspective on the controversy regarding "natural" versus "synthetic" medications.

## *An Overview of Herbal Medicine*

Although the Chinese were early advocates of herbal medicines, they were neither the first, nor the only culture to use herbal medicines. In fact, in the Middle East, India, Egypt, Greece, and Rome, the use of herbal medicines was the primary method of treatment. Even today, it is estimated that that up to 80 percent of the world's population still depends primarily on herbal remedies.

The most common method of delivering these medicines is in the form of tea, although herbal treatments are also given as infusions, decoctions, compresses, or poultices.

An infusion is created by pouring boiling water over an herb or other materials, such as flowers, bark, roots, or berries. A decoction is made by simmering these same materials in water. Compresses are created by soaking a cloth in the liquid produced by an infusion or decoction and applying the cloth to the skin. Poultices are created by applying the fresh herb or other material directly to the body and covering it with a bandage or cloth.

While in Western medicine medications are generally prescribed to treat a specific condition, in Chinese medicine, combinations of herbs are often formulated to cure several things at once. Most Chinese herbs are made into strong teas. (The taste of these teas may at first be difficult to get used to by people who have not grown up with them.)

Most alternative medical systems involve the use of "natural" medicines. While we may tend to associate herbal remedies with Chinese medicine, not all herbal or "natural" remedies actually come from Eastern cultures. Native Americans have a strong healing tradition that includes both the spiritual and religious elements of Eastern medicine as well as a pharmacoepia of herbal medicines. The combination of the spiritual and healing is common to many cultures that use herbal remedies as the basis for treating ailments..

## The Creation of "Synthetic" or "Chemical" Medicines

Americans have depended largely on herbal remedies throughout most of their history, but since the mid-1800s the trend in Western medicine has become increasingly more scientific. Until just over 100 years ago, Americans, since they had no idea what caused infections, didn't even wash their hands or their medical instruments between patients.

Before the discovery of penicillin by Scottish scientist Alexander Fleming in 1928 (first tested on humans in 1941) antibiotics as we know them did not exist. Diseases caused by bacteria like tuberculosis and infections killed thousands of people each year. After antibiotics became available, people who previously would have certainly died from what is considered today a benign infection, were cured within weeks or even days.

A huge medical advance, vaccination against disease, had been made more than a century earlier by Edward Jenner, who developed a vaccine for smallpox in 1798. By the 1930s vaccines had also been developed for rabies, plague, diphtheria, pertussis, tuberculosis, tetanus and yellow fever and in the 1950s and 1960s, vaccines for polio, measles, and mumps. And finally, in the 1970s and early 1980s, vaccines for rubella and hepatitis B.

Other medical breakthroughs included Louis Pasteur's discovery in the mid-1800s that germs caused disease and the discovery of insulin in 1922 by Frederick Banting and Charles Best.

All of these discoveries, combined with the availability of predictably clean water made a tremendous impact on public health. As scientists began to formulate increasingly effective medicines for other ailments, it is little wonder people began to abandon folk cures in favor of the "miracle cures" that kept (and keep) appearing on the market.

By the 1950s, traditional healers and medicines were considered by many to be hopelessly old fashioned and ineffective. The best medicine was medicine created by a pharmaceutical company and the best place for treatment was in a nice clean hospital, complete with a multitude of devices, machines and medicines that were there to "cure" all ailments.

## A Renewed Interest in Herbal Medicines

In the 1960s, however, there was a backlash of sorts. Young adults began to rebel against what they considered the overly materialistic lifestyles of their parents and along with their back-to-a-simpler-life philosophy came a renewed interest in all things natural, including foods and medicines. History and politics at the time had a lot to do with the philosophy that opposed anything fabricated and engi- neered. The natural way became the only real way, unless, of course, you were desperate.

While, as they aged, most 1960s hippies became disillusioned with the harsh realities of subsistence farming and communal lifestyle, many have brought with them into middle age the belief that "natu- ral" foods and medicines are still somehow superior to those pro- duced "chemically." Largely because of this market, as any visit to a natural food store will verify, there are now thousands of "natural" products from which to choose. The trend for all things natural again became not only popular, but also very well marketed!

## The Evolution from "Natural" to Chemical or Synthetic

Since this debate about avoiding "chemical" products is confusing to many people, it deserves some discussion.

First, it should be noted that most medicines that we use today either are or have evolved from "natural" products. Digitalis, for example, is a heart drug that is derived from foxglove, a flowering plant. Lotions made with aloe vera soothe the pain of sunburn, the bark of the yew tree is the source of the cancer drug, Taxol. Anise, often used to stop heartburn, comes from the dried fruit of Pimpinella anisum and is often taken therapeutically in tea.

Throughout history, however, few healers have prescribed "natural" remedies in their natural state.

The first change to most natural remedies was aesthetic. Even the earliest healers realized that a medicine wasn't much good if the patient wouldn't take it. So, since many herbal cures were somewhat less than palatable, healers began to mix these natural substances with alcohol, spices and perfumes and dye them more attractive colors.

As time went on, those formulating medicines also began to address other issues.

The first of these was purity. Even though until the mid 1800s doctors didn't have the faintest idea about what caused infection, they did seem to understand that using "natural" things meant that they were getting a lot of cross contamination. Grinding up a whole Majorana hortensis Moench, for example, produced the desired amount of marjoram but it also contained a small proportion of the flowering tops of the plant.

As they began to understand the chemistry of the substances they were using, they began to be able to isolate just what the desired ingredient was. Once they had isolated it, beginning in most cases in the 1800s, scientists figured out how to produce these medicines "chemically," thus being reliably able to separate out from the natural source just the ingredients they needed.

Another issue was correct dosage. In its "natural" state, the medicinal level of many herbs and other plants is highly unpredictable. Different strains of a plant, or plants grown in different soils may produce a wide variety of different potencies. Without chemical testing, there was no way to be sure except by trial and error. As soon as a drug could be produced chemically, each dose could be assured to be identical.

Another issue was availability and convenience. Medicines were one of the first products to be traded internationally as the first explorers brought back with them the magic potions they had found on their travels. While such drugs were often effective, they were not only expensive to import, but were often difficult to obtain. The ability to produce them synthetically assured a consistent supply.

Yet another issue was direct action. Most botanicals contain not just one but many compounds, which may have a variety of effects. In an effort to cure one problem, another was sometimes created. For example, a certain medicinal tea might work well to fight a fever, but might also be a powerful laxative. Using the herb in its "natural" state, it was impossible to separate the two effects. Isolating the different elements of the drug and finding which produced which effect allowed the drug to work in only the desired way.

Also, herbs in their "natural" state often caused unpleasant side effects because the recipient was allergic to one of the many active ingredients in the remedy. By isolating the desired active ingredient, "synthetic" drugs can be better formulated to eliminate untoward side effects.

And finally, there was the issue of regulation. Throughout most of history, the production of medicines was largely unregulated. The best a patient could hope for was a reputable and competent pharmacist or doctor. If either wasn't reputable or competent, there was little recourse. Since there was no central testing facility, anyone could mix up just about anything and, providing it didn't kill anyone, get by with selling it to the unsuspecting public.

A prime example of this was the traveling "medicine shows" that were big attractions during the 1800s in this country. Although the medicines sold by these itinerant entertainers were usually mostly alcohol, or in some cases cocaine or morphine, the medicine man was out of town days before the patient realized that that happy feeling he got from the drug wasn't doing much to solve the initial problem. Additionally, there was virtually no inspection of drugs, so even efficacious drugs could often be contaminated.

## The Advent of Regulation

The US government began to regulate drugs as early as 1862, with the hiring of a single chemist in the US Department of Agriculture. Prior to this time the regulation of drugs, such as it was, rested with the states. In 1906, the Federal Food and Drugs Act created the modern Food and Drug Administration which, in 1940 was moved to the Federal Security Agency and in 1953 transferred to the Department of Health Education And Welfare, which in 1980 became the Department of Health and Human Services. Now this giant bureaucracy includes more than 9,000 employees and has a budget of more than $1 billion. In addition to approving drugs, the agency also regulates medical devices, food and color additives, infant formula, animal drugs and monitors the manufacture, import, transport, storage and sale of $1 trillion worth of products. (www.fda.gov) Today, all prescription drugs sold by US manufacturers must be approved by the FDA before they may be sold to the public.

## Summary

Gastroenterologists and other medical professionals understand that treatment of disease is a very individual thing. Patients with the same symptoms often respond very differently to the medications and lifestyle changes we recommend. Likewise, some patients may well benefit from some of the complementary or alternative medications or therapies we have discussed in this chapter. Because all medications and therapies have the potential to interact with one another, however, before trying any of these alternative or complementary regimens, I would certainly recommend that you discuss this idea with your doctor. And certainly, if you are now using any of these alternative medications or therapies, you should always tell your doctor, to be sure that anything he or she prescribes will not result in an unpleasant side effect with these other medications.

One major difference between herbal and traditionally prescribed medicines is that herbal therapies are not approved by the US Food and Drug Administration (FDA). According to the FDA, any product is a "drug" if it is "intended for use in the cure, mitigation, treatment, or prevention of disease." Since herbs are not marketed as "drugs," the FDA does not have to approve the agent for distribution, as long as the agent has not proven to be harmful to those who consume the quantities recommended on the packaging.

If an herb is marketed as a drug, in advertisements, magazines, pamphlets, on television, on the internet, or in any other way, the "drug" must be "recognized as safe and effective for the referenced condition" for it to be legally distributed. Dietary supplements, however, can be legally marketed as long as therapeutic claims are removed from promotional materials, otherwise, the sale of the herb will be in violation of FDA regulations and will not be allowed for sale. Since many makers of herbal medicines do not market them as "drugs," they are free from FDA stringent restrictions on distribution. Calling them nutritional supplements makes them a much easier to sell.

As a consumer, it is very important for you to understand this very important distinction between FDA approved and non-FDA approved distribution of medicinal agents. Remember, although the herb may have a long history of helping a particular ailment, or the herb has been touted as the "best" treatment for your condition, it is important to realize that this remedy is unlikely to have undergone the rigorous scrutiny of FDA approval to ensure its safety for that particular use.

This does not mean that the herb will not help you. It only means that the herb, since it has not been approved for medicinal use, is distinctly different in that whoever is selling it has not had to prove that it actually works for the condition you may be using it for. The majority of herbs used have not been formally tested in double-blind placebo-controlled trials, so it is difficult to prove their efficacy as a treatment for disease. Thus, there is a great difference between many herbal remedies and the traditionally prescribed drugs that must undergo such scrutiny, typically lasting several years, to ensure, as much as possible, safety to you as the consumer.

## Unregulated Products

The production of herbal medicinal products in this country remains largely unregulated. The more than 20,000 vitamins, herbs and minerals now on the market are not subject to FDA monitoring. Manufacturers of these products are not required to provide either information about the contents of these compounds or the method of preparation. Unlike other drugs, they are also not required to mention possible side effects or provide any proof of efficacy. Some, like those offered in the old time medicine shows, provide "more desirable" results by the addition of caffeine or alcohol. Most have not been scientifically tested.

In addition to this lack of scrutiny, many of these products are imported from other countries so there is no way of knowing how they were grown, harvested or stored, what pesticides may have been used on them, and if there are additives that will be unknown to the consumer. These are very important concerns for you to be aware of, particularly if you are tempted to purchase herbs from a local herbalist or nutrition store. As a user of herbs be a discriminating buyer and be aware of these important facts.

Also, it should also be noted that "natural" doesn't necessarily mean safe. Some herbs that grow naturally, perhaps even in your own backyard, can be very dangerous to your health. Other herbs may be safe, but completely useless in treating disease or your particular complaint or discomfort.

In addition, because all of these "natural" medicines have some physical effect, they may have a very different or, again dangerous, effect if taken in combination with other natural or synthetic medicines. Although these herbal agents are not technically considered "drugs" by the FDA's definition, they do have the capacity to compete with drugs and other supplements for metabolism and can damage the liver, kidneys or other internal organs, particularly if taken in excess or with other agents, either prescription drugs or supplements. Before you decide to mix various supplements and drugs be sure to consult your physician.

## Food Supplements

Almost every natural food store and many pharmacies and grocery stores now contain a wide variety of food supplements whose manufacturers make many claims about their benefits. For example, many advocates of "natural" foods recommend foods and supplements such as licorice (to coat and protect the esophagus), marshmallow (to coat and protect irritated mucous membranes) and aloe vera (which acts as an anti-inflammatory).

Since every herb has very different potential effects, lack of information does not necessarily equate with a lack of benefit. To use a non-FDA approved supplement, use the options available that are known and proven clinically to work in patients with that ailment (reflux, for example). If all of the known traditional approaches have failed, assuming that there is no evidence to support danger with that particular supplement, carefully select one to see if it works. Sometimes the agent works and sometimes it doesn't. Much of this form of treatment is trial and error since there is little published regarding many of the herbs used at the current time. Since there is little doubt that licorice and marshmallow cause no harm such therapies using these ingredients may be useful. Ideally, however, such recommendations should be supported by clinical data that proves the effectiveness of that agent.

Prior to the initiation of any course of treatment, particularly the use of any alternative therapies, consult your primary physician or gastroenterologist.

In summary, be wary of any supplement or herbal remedy that you try or that others recommend to you. Although not labeled as "drugs," they can certainly act like drugs in that they may have side effects, interactions and effects on internal organs such as the kidney, liver, pancreas, thyroid gland, among others that can be harmful to your health.

Supplements are probably not necessary for the average person who eats a well balanced diet. Food supplements sometimes are recommended to those who are nutritionally deficient because of underlying medical problems such as alcoholism, patients with a large amount of surgical intestinal resection, patients with liver disease or patients prone to osteoporosis, and patients who are limited in their diet, such as vegans and vegetarians. Although these are a few examples of the type of patients that may need supplements, they a minority of the population. If you eat a healthy, well balanced diet, you probably don't need to take supplements!

## Digestive Enzymes

In addition to food supplements, many health food stores also offer digestive enzymes. Digestive enzymes are proteins that act as catalysts for the various biological and chemical reactions in the body, including digestion. Most of these enzymes are naturally produced throughout the digestive tract, beginning in the mouth (there are enzymes in saliva) and ending in the large intestine. These enzymes include amylase, lipase, protease, lactase, bromelain and papain.

It is important to note that there is no conclusive evidence that enzyme supplements help patients without known diseases of the digestive tract such as chronic pancreatitis, or patients with a history of surgical resection of the pancreas or stomach. Physicians do not typically recommend these enzymes to patients without known problems relating to their pancreas or digestive tract.

Still, the majority of people who take these remedies are not those with known significant pancreatic or digestive disease, but, rather, are patients who believe they do not digest appropriately. There is no good clinical data to support that these agents significantly improve digestion, particularly if there is no digestive organ disease. Most physicians typically do not advise their patients to take such supplements to merely "help" their digestion, as there is no good evidence to support that this actually occurs.

On the one hand, these supplements typically cause no harm and are not harmful to others. On the other hand, it is doubtful if you will derive any benefit from them. Before you try any of these enzymes or supplements, I would highly recommend that you begin a regimen centered on dietary and lifestyle change. These changes are far more likely to relieve the symptoms you are experiencing and will certainly cost you less than experimenting with a variety of health food store products.

# 13

# SURGICAL OPTIONS
## *An Overview*

P EOPLE HAVE BEEN TAKING VARIOUS MEDICATIONS for GERD for centuries. Unfortunately for some, no matter what they took or even how faithful they were about watching their diets, many continued to suffer frequent and severe episodes of GERD. For many, surgery became the only option.

In this chapter we review the advantages and disadvantages of surgery as treatment for GERD. We also discuss the surgical options available to those for whom medication alone has provided no relief.

## *When is Surgery Recommended?*

Because surgery of any kind presents a certain amount of risk, expense, and discomfort, most gastroenterologists recommend surgery only as a last resort and after both medication and endoscopic treatment have failed or been ruled out for other reasons. Surgery should become an option only after pH and motility studies have indicated that reflux is indeed the problem. If motility is abnormal or there is no evidence of reflux, surgery will not help. It is also important, of course, to rule out any other cause for the symptoms before proceeding with surgery—particularly with surgical procedures that are irreversible.

Still, for some people, the risks, discomfort, and expense of surgery may be well worth it.

In general, surgery is recommended for the following:

PEOPLE YOUNGER THAN 50 YEARS OF AGE  GERD can occur in people of all ages. When a person 50 years old or younger suffers from recurrent and frequent GERD, surgery is sometimes recommended to forestall decades of potential complications such as Barrett's esophagus, strictures, esophagitis, and ulceration.

PEOPLE WITH CHRONIC GERD.  The frequency with which GERD occurs is of major concern because of the damage it can do. Because many GERD medications are comparatively new and lack data about their long-term use, patients sometimes elect to have surgery, hoping that it will eliminate their reliance on medication.

It is true that in the case of H2 blockers and PPIs there are no data documenting the effects of long-term use. However, it is important to remember that there are no known documented cases of cancers or other serious problems believed to be caused by taking these medications.

PEOPLE WITH BARRETT'S ESOPHAGUS OR HIGH-GRADE DYSPLASIA. In some patients, GERD has been treated for long enough and with such poor results that there is an imminent threat of esophageal cancer. In those cases, we sometimes recommend surgery to try to reduce acid reflux into the esophagus. We may even need to consider more than one type of surgery. It is important to note that while surgery may be beneficial, there is no evidence that surgery *prevents* progression from Barrett's esophagus to esophageal cancer. Therefore, even if surgery is performed, we will always recommend that surveil-

lance endoscopy be continued. Another option may be to continue
to use drug therapy but to do regular surveillance endoscopies with
biopsies to make sure there is no new transition to cancer.

PATIENTS WITH LARGE HIATAL HERNIAS   Hernias seldom become
smaller on their own and in morbidly obese patients they can often
enlarge considerably. And hernias are often unaffected by lifestyle
changes or medication. When we determine that a large hernia is the
primary or secondary cause of GERD, the only solution may be to
repair it surgically. As we mention later in this chapter, a Nissen fundoplication procedure is often combined with a hernia repair.

PATIENTS WITH SEVERE COMPLICATIONS OF GERD   Patients who
have severe complications often suffer from more than one problem.
In these instances, it is important to evaluate the situation and decide
which surgical approach, if any, is the most appropriate.

PATIENTS WHO NEED INCREASING OR VERY HIGH DOSES OF MED-
ICATION   Although some medications may work well, physicians
become concerned if a patient seems to require an ever increasing
amount of medication to gain relief, since sooner or later this patient
will no doubt begin to experience some uncomfortable side effects.
Thus, at this point, surgery may be the best option.

PATIENTS WHO SUFFER SIDE EFFECTS FROM MEDICATIONS OR ARE
UNABLE TO TOLERATE THE MEDICATIONS THAT ARE NOW AVAILABLE
Even if a medication works well, if the side effects are severe, we may
recommend surgery instead of continuing a course of medication.
    Again, however, it is important to stress that surgery is rarely nec-
essary. The first options are always weight loss, lifestyle change, antacid
or other medication use and stress reduction.

## *What Are The Advantages of Surgery?*

SURGERY MAY ELIMINATE THE NEED FOR MEDICATION.  There are certainly exceptions, but for most people, surgery either eliminates the need for medication or lessens the required dosage. Surgery is also an advantage for people who do not like to, or cannot remember to take their medication.

SURGERY USUALLY STOPS THE PROGRESSION OF THE DISEASE.  As we have discussed in earlier chapters, most GERD sufferers can manage the disease successfully through dietary and lifestyle changes or with medication. Other people gain no relief from those measures. For them, surgery may allow them to reduce the effect of acid injury on the esophagus secondary to reflux.

SURGERY MAY PREVENT THE LONG-TERM EFFECTS OF GERD.  As we have mentioned above, if a GERD sufferer is very young or seems to have frequent episodes of GERD, sooner or later he or she will probably suffer some long-term effects. Surgery may offer relief that was not achievable through medical or endoscopic therapy.

SURGERY MAY BE THE MOST COST-EFFECTIVE OPTION  In some cases, surgery is covered by a patient's insurance while medications, particularly over-the-counter medications, are not. In the long run, surgery becomes less expensive than medication.

## *What Are the Disadvantages of Surgery?*

HOSPITAL STAYS OF VARYING LENGTHS. For invasive surgical proce-dures, a hospital stay of up to a week and a recovery period of up to eight weeks is likely. For minimally invasive surgeries (as in laparo-scopic Nissen fundoplication repair or laparoscopic hiatal hernia repair), the hospital stay may be two to three days and the recovery period a couple of weeks or so.

UNCOMFORTABLE AFTEREFFECTS.  Many patients experience flatulence and bloating or abdominal discomfort for several days following surgery. This is because surgery temporarily affects intestinal function. Typically, as complete healing occurs, normal intestinal function resumes and the bloating and flatulence cease.

Chronic dysphagia is a condition that can result from surgery, although it occurs in less than 5 percent of patients. It is usually the result of a wrap that was made too tight. In these patients the symptoms may occur chronically, that is, repeatedly over time. These patients may also lose the ability to vomit. Some patients opt for reversal surgery to correct this undesirable situation.

TEMPORARY DIETARY RESTRICTIONS.  Because the stomach is involved in the surgery, patients will probably be restricted to liquid or soft foods for a period of several days or occasionally for even a few weeks.

POSSIBLE (MINOR) SCARRING.  The scarring resulting from an open Nissen fundoplication is usually six to 10 inches long.

RISK OF COMPLICATIONS.  Any surgery that requires an incision, external or internal, presents a risk of post-operative infections. And anytime anesthetic or any kind of sedation is used, there is risk (albeit small) of cardiac or pulmonary complications, particularly among very ill or very old patients.

SURGERY IS NOT APPROPRIATE FOR ALL PATIENTS.  Although most patients and surgeons are now able to take advantage of the less invasive laparoscopic procedures, those procedures might not be appropriate for a small number of patients. Moreover, some patients are poor candidates for any kind of surgery, even the most minimally invasive. These patients would include the morbidly obese, patients with a multitude of co-existing medical problems and those at risk for any kind of surgery including those with diabetes or heart disease.

SURGERY DOESN'T ALWAYS ELIMINATE THE NEED FOR MEDICATION. Even if the surgery is successful, at least some medication may still be required. A study in the May 9, 1999, edition of *The Journal of American Medical Association* showed that 62 percent of people who underwent surgery to treat GERD still needed medications to manage their condition 10 years later. It is important to note, however, that the interpretation of this study is the subject of some controversy because the subjects were residents at a veterans hospital. Therefore, the results may not be applicable to the majority of patients undergoing this surgery. There is also literature to support the fact that after a laparoscopic Nissen, patients have as low as a 14 percent incidence of requiring medicines after surgery when evaluated at a seven-year follow up.

SOME SURGERIES MAY NEED TO BE REPEATED. This is particularly true of those in which the procedure resulted in the opening to the stomach being too large or too small.

Because the end of the esophagus may be mildly inflamed following surgery, the patient may experience the sensation of food getting stuck in the throat. When the swelling diminishes, however, this symptom typically disappears.

## Surgery Options for GERD Sufferers

NISSEN FUNDOPLICATION. Many types of surgery have been attempted through the ages and surgery as we know it (using anesthetics and sterile techniques) became an option for sufferers of many diseases as early as the late 1800s. But it wasn't until the early 1950s, thanks to Dr. Frederick Nissen, that surgery became available as a treatment for GERD.

Since the problem faced by most GERD patients was an ineffective LES, Dr. Nissen reasoned that the problem could be solved by wrapping the top of the stomach (known as the gastric fundus) around the lower portion of the esophagus. This surgical procedure, named after its inventor, is called the Nissen Fundoplication. Although the procedure does not replace the faulty LES, it does create a mechanical barrier that prevents the flow of acid up the esophagus. This procedure is often combined with a repair of a hiatal hernia.

The Nissen fundoplication is an invasive procedure. General anesthesia is administered and the surgeon makes a six- to 10-inch incision in the middle of the abdomen, from just below the ribs to the belly button. The chest is "cracked" and several bones broken. The surgery itself takes from one to three hours. After surgery, the patient is generally required to stay in the hospital for up to a week; total recovery usually takes six to eight weeks. The patient is also left with a six- to 10-inch surgical scar. In contrast to this type of surgery there is a newer laparoscopic procedure, which we discuss below.

Although the Nissen fundoplication does pose some risks to the patient, as does any surgery, it works so well that it was the just about the only surgical procedure used to treat GERD for nearly 40 years. In some instances it remains the preferred surgery. Some reports suggest that up to 90 percent of patients who have the operation experience at least temporary relief, and many no longer need to take medication of any kind for their heartburn. However, more recent literature casts doubt on this percentage and suggests decreased long-term success for the surgery.

LAPAROSCOPIC NISSEN FUNDOPLICATION. In the early 1990s, a less invasive procedure for fundoplication was developed by a Belgian physician, Dr. Bernard Dallemange. Dallemange's procedure accomplishes the same result as Dr. Nissen's, but the technique is quite different. A long tube called a trocar is inserted into the abdomen through a tiny incision. A laparoscope (an instrument with a tiny video camera mounted on one end) is then fed through the trocar to the site of the procedure. Since the surgeon can't directly see the site of the surgery, he or she depends on the magnified images transmitted by the laparoscope to a large video monitor.

After the laparoscope is in position, four other trocars are inserted through more tiny incisions surrounding the site of the surgery. These other trocars are used for the surgical instruments required for the operation. The abdomen is also inflated with carbon dioxide to give the surgeon more room to work.

During the operation, the surgeon first pulls back the liver to expose the site of the surgery. Next, he or she then clamps the blood vessels around the site, positions the top of the stomach around the end of the esophagus, and sutures it in place. Once the operation is complete, the trocars are removed and each incision is closed. Because the trocar incisions are so small, they require only a stitch or two and are generally covered with a small bandage.

A laparoscopic fundoplication generally takes about an hour and a half to two hours. It, too, requires a general anesthetic, but since the surgery is minimally invasive, the hospital stay is relatively short, usually between one to two days. Afterward, a full recovery is made within two weeks. The surgical scars—which are about a centimeter long—usually disappear within a few months.

In occasional (but rare) instances, laparoscopic fundoplication cannot be completed as planned and the surgeon must perform a Nissen fundoplication instead.

TOUPET PARTIAL FUNDOPLICATION, HILL REPAIR, AND BELSEY MARK IV. Three other surgical techniques—Toupet Partial Fundoplication, Hill Repair, and Belsey Mark IV—are also used to treat GERD, although not nearly as commonly as the Nissen fundoplication. In these surgeries, the LES is actually restructured to improve its strength. The major differences between the Hill Repair and the Belsey procedures is that the Hill Repair is done from below the diaphragm and the Belsey is done from above the diaphragm. The Toupet Partial fundoplication is a partial posterior fundoplication. It is usually done also from below the diaphragm. This procedure can also be done laparoscopically.

These procedures are done on an inpatient basis. The patient can expect to stay two to seven days in the hospital and fully recover in two to six weeks.

LAPAROSCOPIC HIATAL HERNIA REPAIR.  Hiatal hernia is a condition in which part of the stomach has protruded through the diaphragm and into the hiatus, the opening into the chest. If a hiatal hernia becomes large enough to exert pressure on the LES or causes upper GI symptoms and reflux into the esophagus, it may need to be repaired surgically. This is also a laparoscopic outpatient procedure in which the surgeon inserts trocars into small incisions in the abdomen, one containing the laparoscope and the other surgical instruments.

Since the problem is that a part of the stomach has protruded through the hiatus (the opening into the chest), the purpose of the surgery is to strengthen the hiatus, so that the upper part of the stomach can no longer get through it. To do this, the surgeon sews the opening closed around the esophagus.  Patients undergoing Nissen Fundlopications often require a hiatal hernia repair as well.

Generally the patient can go home the day after the surgery or within a few days. Recovery time is typically two to three weeks.

SURGICAL MYOTOMY (CARDIOMYOTOMY).  While most surgeries for GERD or the results of GERD are focused on making the junction of the stomach and esophagus smaller, in instances where the patient suffers from achalasia (a condition in which the LES fails to relax), an operation called a cardiomyotomy is sometimes performed. In this surgery, some of the muscles at the entrance to the stomach are cut to enlarge the passageway for food to enter the stomach.

Note that in this case the prefix *cardio* refers to the cardia, the upper portion of the stomach, and not the heart. *Myotomy* means "cutting a muscle surgically."

While surgery is certainly an option in treating GERD, it is very important that you weigh all the advantages and disadvantages before you choose to undergo a surgical procedure. Be sure to consult not only with your doctor but also a surgeon to make sure you understand all that may be involved. Also make sure that your surgeon is experienced in doing the procedure you are anticipating.

# 14

# LIFESTYLE CHANGES
## *Steps You Can Take Today*

IN ADDITION TO THE MANY OPTIONS WE HAVE discussed in earlier chapters, achieving long-term relief from GERD also involves some fundamental lifestyle change for most people. Although we have mentioned several of these changes before, here's a rundown of the steps you can take to relieve GERD symptoms.

## *Stop Smoking*

Of all the things you can change about your current lifestyle, if you are a smoker, stopping is probably the most important. Nearly 500,000 people die each year from diseases related to smoking and your risk of developing lung cancer is 10 times greater than if you were a non-smoker. If you are now smoking two packs of cigarettes a day, that risk rises to 15 to 25 percent. If you suffer from GERD, your risks are even higher since the smoke you draw into your esophagus further irritates tissue that may already be inflamed, not to mention that smoking is also a predictive factor for esophageal cancer.

It is not easy to quit smoking (of the 17 million Americans who try annually, only about 1.3 million actually succeed, according to FDA publication 94-3203). But we urge you in the strongest terms to become one of those 1.3 million. It may not only save your life but it will also decrease the likelihood of developing GERD, cancers of the airway or digestive tract, and bad breath, to mention a few.

There are now many products and programs available to help you. The most widely used products are transdermal patches and smoking cessation chewing gum. These products contain nicotine (one of the more than 4,000 chemicals in cigarettes) that most researchers agree results in addiction. Patches and chewing gum work by replacing the nicotine from cigarettes in gradually diminishing amounts until you no longer feel the need for it.

Although many people find that the patch or chewing gum is enough, many other people greatly benefit from counseling or a smoking cessation program, as well. Such programs not only provide emotional support to you as you withdraw from the nicotine, but also help you learn to eliminate the habits associated with smoking. Your doctor can recommend programs in your area.

## Avoid Lying Down Right After a Heavy Meal or Snack

If you suffer frequently from GERD, chances are that you have a weakened or malfunctioning LES. Just after a meal, your stomach produces acid and contracts and expands. This process exerts pressure on this valve and in your case, can easily result in acid being refluxed into your esophagus. You can help prevent this from happening by remaining upright by standing or sitting since the force of gravity will help to keep the food and acid where it belongs. If you lie down, however, you face a much greater risk that your weakened LES will not be able to counteract the pressure in the stomach and at least a portion of what is in your stomach will reflux back into your esophagus.

Another important causal factor is the size of the meal. No matter how well your LES works, if you put enough food in your stomach to expand it greatly, you can add to the stretch pressure exerted from the stomach to the LES, again weakening the valve and keeping it from closing properly. Since digestion takes time, we recommend that you remain upright for at least two or three hours after a meal or heavy snack. I would also recommend that rather than eating three large meals a day, that you eat 5-6five to six smaller portion meals a day.

### After Eating, Avoid Vigorous Exercise or Any Activity that Requires Stooping or Bending Over

Vigorous exercise or anything that requires stooping or bending over right after eating can cause reflux to just about anybody. If you regularly experience GERD, your chances of this happening are greatly increased. The problem, again, is that the digesting food is already exerting pressure on your LES. When you add additional pressure by squeezing the midsection of your body, reflux is a common result. Major causes of this are bending over at the gym, extreme Yoga positions (body contortions, bending), power lifting and extreme running.

### Avoid Going to Bed Until Several Hours After a Heavy Meal or Snack

The same problems that are caused by lying down, exercising or bending over after eating a meal or a heavy snack are only increased if you go to bed. There are several reasons for this.

First, by lying even flatter than you might if you were lying on the couch watching television, you give gravity even less chance to help your LES keep the food in the stomach as it is being digested.

Second, if you generally depend on an antacid to relieve symptoms of GERD, it will only work so long. If you go to bed immediately after a heavy meal, the antacid will work for awhile, but since digestion takes many hours, symptoms of GERD may well wake you from sleep. This is exacerbated not only by new acid production in the stomach in response to food, but also by the effect gravity has on the acid contents of the stomach flowing into the esophagus.

## Eliminate or Decrease Your Intake of Alcoholic Beverages

In addition to providing "empty" calories, alcoholic beverages often increase the production of stomach acid and, like cigarette smoke, can irritate the already inflamed tissues that line your esophagus as well as reducing LES pressure. While an occasional glass of wine will probably do you little harm and, indeed, may have some cardiovascular benefit, try to make consumption of alcohol an occasional, not regular part of your lifestyle. Remember, too, that beer and sparkling wines like champagne are not only alcoholic but are also carbonated and that carbonation can cause a build up of gas in the stomach that can, in turn, result in GERD. The same is true of mixers for liquor such as club soda or ginger ale.

If you find that you cannot decrease your intake of alcohol, this may be an early warning sign that you may be suffering from alcoholism. If this is the case, ask your doctor to recommend a program such as Alcoholics Anonymous.

## Exercise More

As I mentioned in Chapter 9, some forms of vigorous exercise can cause GERD in some people. However, the benefits of a sensible and consistent exercise program far outweigh the risks for just about everyone from small children to very elderly people. Take time to reread Chapter 9 and decide which form of exercise would best fit into your new and healthier lifestyle. If you are not physically active at this time, it is also a good idea to have a thorough physical examination before you start to make sure that your heart is healthy and there are no other physical limitations to your new exercise regimen.

## Elevate the Head of Your Bed Several Inches

Many people who suffer from GERD find that they are awakened in the middle of the night with its symptoms. While often this occurs because the effects of the antacid they are taking have simply worn off, sometimes the problem is that when the LES relaxes, it is easier for acid to reflux into the esophagus if you are lying down. Propping yourself up with several pillows will not solve this problem and, in fact, may actually make the situation worse since propping pillows can cause your body to bend forward putting more pressure on your stomach.

Placing wooden blocks under the headboard is a much better solution, as this raises your head and increases the angle of the bed without causing additional pressure on the abdomen. The angle that works best tends to be an individual thing. If you attempt to do this, you should experiment with blocks of different sizes until you find what works best for you.

### *Maintain an Appropriate Weight for Your Age and Height.*

In addition to changing your diet to eliminate those foods that cause GERD for you, if your weight is above the range suggested on the chart on page 79, definitely consider a weight loss program. As we discussed in Chapter 8, dieting for weight loss is a long long-term commitment and should be accomplished slowly and deliberately to avoid the inevitable return to overweight that results from the kinds of quick losses that occur with fad diets. The secret of weight loss is simple. To lose weight, you must expend more calories than you take in. You can only do this through eating less and/or exercising more. A one-step-at-a-time approach in my view is most desirable. Although it may take a little longer for you to lose weight, the process is more reasonable and gradual which in my view is essential for continued compliance with the weight loss regimen. If you need to lose weight, ask your doctor to recommend a weight loss diet or weight loss program in your community.

# 15

# LONG TERM EFFECTS
## *What You Need to Know*

FOR SOME PEOPLE, GERD IS A SHORT-TERM, occasional problem. Something they ate or something they did caused an episode that either went away by itself or was alleviated by an over-the-counter antacid. For others, GERD is a long-term problem that can be sporadic or chronic and persistent. Those who have sporadic GERD may have episodes a few times a month. Over many years they generally find relief from ordinary antacids. For some people, GERD is not only a long-term problem, but also a chronic one. Year after year GERD occurs on a frequent basis, several times a week, or even several times a day. Occasional GERD causes few long-term effects, but chronic, frequent GERD can lead to serious, long-lasting effects. If you are a chronic GERD sufferer, you must learn to be careful about what you eat and the lifestyle choices you make. You should also seek close follow up from your doctor.

Here are some of problems found in patients with chronic GERD.

## *Tooth Decay*

Many people suffering from chronic GERD can have a significant amount of tooth decay. Why? The digestive enzymes in the saliva are mild in comparison to the hydrochloric acid produced in the stomach. The tooth enamel is certainly strong enough to resist saliva, but is often no match for the hydrochloric acid that is refluxed into the esophagus when recurrent episode of GERD occur.

With each episode of GERD, the hydrochloric acid eats away at the tooth enamel, eventually allowing bacteria to enter the tooth and cause decay.

## Halitosis (Bad Breath)

Although certainly unpleasant for the people around you, halitosis, or bad breath, is a good thing, in that it can be an early warning that something is wrong somewhere else in your body. Sometimes the unpleasant odor is simply a result of something you ate. The aromas of very spicy or strong smelling foods can often be absorbed into your circulatory system and released into the lungs and then breathed out as you exhale. This type of halitosis is usually very temporary, lasting less than 24 hours. It does not usually become chronic halitosis.

Smokers and alcoholics also often have halitosis, although theirs tends to be more chronic since they are constantly flooding their mouths with smoke and alcohol. These patients not only have halitosis, but may also have poor dental hygiene with staining, decay, and gum disease in addition to their underlying increased risk of cancer.

Sometimes, halitosis is a result of a problem in your mouth, such as failure to brush your teeth correctly, failure to floss regularly or poorly maintained dentures. In these cases, the cause of the odor is usually bacterial growth caused by food remaining in between the teeth. Other times, halitosis is a symptom of an infection such as those caused by gum disease or tooth decay. A fever of any kind may also produce halitosis.

GERD is also a frequent cause of halitosis, since the food that refluxes up the esophagus from the stomach is only partially digested and food in general, if left to sit anywhere (in the stomach and esophagus, for instance) will often become malodorous. In the case of

GERD, the odor is typically caused by stagnant food.

Trying to mask the odor with breath mints for halitosis may work temporarily, but in most cases the only way it will be eliminated will be by treating the underlying problem. In the case of GERD, breath mints may actually cause the problem to get worse, since mint can relax the LES and allow even more food to reflux into the esophagus.

## Cherry Donner Syndrome (Reflux Laryngitis)

The larynx, (the voice box) can also be affected by GERD. And because GERD is often chronic, so, too, may be the laryngitis. Because the larynx is a tube—like the esophagus—it is lined with epithelial cells which, when irritated may become inflamed. Common symptoms of laryngitis are hoarseness, loss of voice or soreness. Laryngitis is also caused by infection, smoking, excessive alcohol use or shouting. Laryngitis or a hoarse voice may be an indicator of chronic GERD, particularly if there is also an associated chronic cough.

## Long-Term Effects in the Esophagus

Most of the problems caused by GERD, however, occur in the esophagus and, because of the chronic nature of GERD, problems in the esophagus may go from bad to worse fairly quickly. That is why it is so important for you to seek the advice of a doctor if the GERD you are experiencing occurs on more than a very occasional basis.

The following diseases of the esophagus are common among GERD sufferers.

REFLUX ESOPHAGITIS.    Those who experience GERD on a chronic basis almost always eventually suffer from reflux esophagitis, a condition in which the cells of the esophagus become inflamed causing redness and soreness.

Reflux esophagitis is the most common consequence of GERD (other than pain) and can be mild, moderate, or severe. Reflux esophagitis is typically found by endoscopy and is characterized by the gastro-esophageal junction (also known as the z-line) becoming irregular, inflamed, or ulcerated. Reflux esophagitis can easily be diagnosed by finding erosions (red marks with some blood, as if someone took a sandpaper to the esophagus) at the z-line, swelling, or even ulcerations. If there is a question of this diagnosis, a biopsy of this area can easily distinguish between normal and reflux esophagitis. Esophagitis patients typically have cells called eosinophils in the tissue biopsy if they have esophagitis. Worsening reflux can actually cause ulcers.

EROSIVE ESOPHAGITIS. If left untreated, erosive esophagitis, a more severe form of reflux esophagitis, can occur. In this condition, the mucosa (the surface layers of cells that line the esophagus) are worn away causing erosions, or a superficial irritation or ulceration. A scrape like appearance of the tissue is typically found in patients with erosive esophagitis. It is most commonly found at the distal end of the esophagus; however it can also occur along the entire length. The result is a severe burning sensation and/or pain behind the breastbone spreading into the shoulders, neck and/or face. Not surprisingly, this condition is often mistaken for a heart attack. Other symptoms of erosive esophagitis include nausea, difficulty in swallowing, the feeling that food won't go down and persistent cough. In severe cases, bleeding may occur.

ULCERATIVE ESOPHAGITIS. In addition to the wearing away of the mucosa, if GERD is allowed to continue to occur, ulcers can also form on the wall of the esophagus. Ulcerative esophagitis is a condition that is just one step more serious than erosive esophagitis. The main difference is that an ulcer (or ulcers) is clearly visible, however the same symptoms mentioned earlier still apply. Ulcerative esophagitis is more likely to cause bleeding into the intestinal tract. Sometimes the bleeding can be quite severe. Ulcerative esophagitis responds quite well to proton pump inhibitor. Many patients with ulcerative esophagitis feel much better after an eight-week course of a PPI.

STRICTURE OF THE ESOPHAGUS.   If the esophagus is allowed to be inflamed long enough, eventually reflux can cause an accumulation of scar tissue and the scarring in turn can cause a gradual narrowing of the esophagus. The inevitable result is difficulty in swallowing. This condition is called dysphagia.

Two main types of scarring are thought to be caused by the effect of reflux on the esophagus. One is the formation of what is called a Schatzki's ring. This is a scar that forms a ring, often one that is non-obstructing, just at the gastro-esophageal junction, or the z-line. This "ring" is a fibrous scar or thickening that, although it is completely benign (not pre-cancerous) can cause significant episodes of dysphagia.

If food gets stuck in this ring (typically after eating quickly without enough water) the patient can experience intense pain. There can be a complete obstruction of the esophagus and an inability to keep ones secretions down. This often leads to an emergency room visit with persistent pain and "spitting up" saliva. If not treated, this scarring can result in esophageal ulceration and further scarring.

Treatment consists of an emergency endoscopy and removal of the obstructing foreign body. Once the foreign body is removed, the symptoms almost immediately abate. The patient should then consider elective upper endoscopy to "dilate" the ring. Often, esophageal dilations can be performed in the doctor's office. Although there is a slight risk of perforation of the esophagus, most patients tolerate the procedure well without any serious consequences. Occasionally these rings come back and patients may need a repeat dilation.

Esophageal strictures have the same symptoms as rings and can also cause food impaction and dysphagia. The difference is that these strictures are more likely to be longer bands of scarring rather than rings. Strictures are treated the same way as rings since a stricture can be a thicker band of scar tissue. Dilation of strictures is typically more difficult than rings and, in general, there is a higher recurrence rate.

NOTE: It is important when diagnosed with a stricture to make sure your gastroenterologist has biopsied the area prior to dilation because some cancers of the esophagus can actually look to the doctor like a stricture with a food impaction or dysphagia.

BARRETT'S ESOPHAGUS AND ADENOCARCINOMA. Barrett's esophagus and adenocarcinoma are two other frequent long term effects of GERD. Since they are both common and very serious, they will be discussed in greater detail in the following chapter.

# 16

# BARRETT'S ESOPHAGUS & CANCER

## *Are You at Risk?*

IN MANY CASES, THE SYMPTOMS OF GERD CAN BE alleviated through changes in diet, lifestyle modification, and medications. When those with GERD symptoms fail to change their diet or lifestyle or take proper medications, the result can be serious. Untreated GERD often leads to a condition called Barrett's esophagus, which can lead to painful cancers that are often fatal.

### Barrett's Esophagus

For reasons not completely understood, about 10 to 15 percent of GERD patients develop Barrett's esophagus, a condition first described by British surgeon Norman Barrett more than 50 years ago. At the time Barrett discovered this condition it was considered fairly benign. However, now we understand that it must be managed carefully by a gastroenterologist since in some patients Barrett's esophagus may develop into esophageal cancer.

Although there is a clear association between Barrett's esophagus and chronic acid reflux, there is no clear-cut recommendation regarding surveillance of the esophagus with upper endoscopy in those who have chronic reflux. In fact, some patients may have reflux for many years and never develop Barrett's esophagus or cancer, while others with chronic reflux may eventually develop Barrett's *and* cancer. Although controversial, many gastroenterologists and esophagologists believe that those who have experienced GERD symptoms for more than five years are more likely to develop Barrett's. Although women and non-Caucasians can certainly develop Barrett's esophagus, it is primarily a disease of white men. Most develop the condition around age 40, but many are not diagnosed with the condition until they are in their 60s. In my practice, I have diagnosed Barrett's in patients as young as their late 20s and as old as 88. This reflects the fact that it can occur at any age; however, the majority of patients are diagnosed between the ages of 30 to 60 decades. These numbers may change in the era of increased evaluation for such conditions, given the current interest and research in this area. Because not everyone with Barrett's esophagus develops cancer, many people with Barrett's esophagus are never diagnosed[1]

CAUSES.  Barrett's esophagus results from severe injury to the squamous epithelium, the cells that line the esophagus. When these cells are injured, generally by the acid that has refluxed up from the stomach, the body attempts to replace these cells, which are not designed to tolerate stomach acid. But the cells are not replaced with similar cells; in fact, the body replaces them with columnar epithelial cells, which are found normally in the intestines and which are designed to tolerate acid. This process is called metaplasia. While this at first seems like the perfect solution to the problem, it is not. We now know that these cells can become dysplastic. That is, these cells can begin to reproduce abnormally and can become cancerous.

Untreated or severe GERD is the primary cause of Barrett's esophagus. Other factors, such as smoking and alcohol consumption, are also considered major factors in the development of this condition, as well as the increased risk of laryngeal or esophageal carcinoma.

Another contributing factor may be duodenogastroesophageal reflux. A subset of people who have severe GERD, including patients with Barrett's esophagus, experience increased back-washing of bile into the esophagus. That condition, called duodenogastroesophageal reflux, occurs when contents from the duodenum (namely bile that is secreted into the duodenum from the liver) refluxes from the duodenum into the stomach, and then from the stomach into the esophagus. This condition is thought to potentially contribute to damage that occurs in patients with barrett's esophagus. Multiple studies, including a study performed in 1997[2], revealed that patients with short segment Barrett's esophagus had an increased prevalence of esophageal bilirubin exposure. The bilirubin detected in the esophagus tended to increase with the degree of esophageal mucosal injury. In fact, the exposure of the esophagus to bilirubin was even higher in patients with longer segments of Barrett's esophagus. Although the mechanism of esophageal injury is not entirely clear, the pancreatic enyzme trypsin and unconjugated bile salts from the duodenum are suspected to be the cause of mucosal damage to the esophagus. Although acid plays a primary role in the development of Barrett's esophagus, there is evidence that bile reflux may contribute to the development of Barrett's esophagus and possibly esophageal adenocarcinoma. The bile reflux is thought to be additive to the effect of acid injury to the esophagus.

Another factor has been thought to be the presence of Helicobacter pylori (H pylori) infection in the stomach, which can cause cancer of the stomach. However recent studies have suggested that H pylori may in fact have a protective effect against the development of Barrett's esophagus by preventing the development of reflux esophagitis which can, in turn, result in Barrett's esophagus and esophageal adenocarcinoma[3]. There is currently much research effort being placed on trying to identify the link that H. Pylori may actually have to acid injury to the esophagus. This is currently under intense investigation.

Increased production of the enzyme cyclooxygenase-2 (COX-2) may also contribute to Barrett's esophagus and the risk of malignancy. This finding has led to the recent suggestion that inhibitors of COX-2 may have a protective effect on the esophagus, thereby potentially preventing the formation of Barrett's esophagus and it's potential transformation to cancer. Current Cox-2 research has shown a potentially protective effect of Cox-2 inhibitor therapy on the esophagus. There is currently, however, no formal FDA approval for the use of Cox-2 inhibitor therapy in patients with Barrett's esophagus.

## Symptoms

Because Barrett's esophagus is generally caused by GERD, the symptoms are similar if not identical, including chest pain, sour mouth, heartburn, persistent cough, and throat pain. Other symptoms may be dysphagia or a sensation that food is stuck in the esophagus, although this typically occurs in the setting of reflux stricture formation or nodule formation with or without dysplasia.

DIAGNOSIS. Since the symptoms of Barrett's esophagus are similar to those of ordinary GERD, it can be specifically diagnosed only by endoscopy. As discussed in Chapter 5, an endoscopy is a procedure in which the gastroenterologist inserts an endoscope, (a long tube with a tiny camera attached) into the esophagus and takes a firsthand look at the esophageal tissue. If the gastroenterologist thinks that the condition may have progressed to cancer, a small sample of the esophageal tissue is taken by the endoscope (called a biopsy) and a pathologist then reviews this tissue under a microscope to identify whether or not there are cancer cells present, Barrett's esophagus, or esophagitis (inflammation without Barrett's type cells or cancer cells).

Because many patients with GERD also have erosive esophagitis, the gastroenterologist may wish to treat it with medications, such as proton pump inhibitors for a period of time. An endoscopy can easily delineate the difference between Barrett's esophagus, erosive esophagitis and other findings such as cancer, in the esophagus. The visual inspection (by viewing through the endoscope alone) is often a strong indicator of the diagnosis, however a biopsy with review by a pathologist is the definitive diagnostic modality. Conditions such as erosive esophagitis respond very well to acid suppression, with medicines such as proton pump inhibitors. Maintenance of these medicines for patients with Barrett's are suggested primarily to prevent progression of the disease, however regression of Barrett's esophagus appears to be unlikely in the majority of cases.

TREATMENT. If a patient has been diagnosed with Barrett's esophagus, modifications in diet and lifestyle are recommended and medications may be prescribed. However, because Barrett's esophagus has the potential to lead to cancer of the esophagus, one of the surgical techniques described in Chapter 13 may be recommended.

What is absolutely essential for a person with Barrett's is to see a gastroenterologist on a regular basis, for at least a second endoscopy in the same year for confirmation of the diagnosis and for more intense tissue sampling. If the diagnosis is clear, surveillance endoscopies are typically performed every one to five years depending on the extent of the Barrett's diagnosis. Most patients will see their gastroenterologist at least three to four times a year to monitor symptoms and to ensure compliance with medical treatment. It is very important that the gastroenterologist monitor the condition closely to make sure that the Barrett's esophagus has not progressed to cancer.

## Laryngeal Carcinoma

Laryngeal carcinoma is cancer of the larynx (voicebox), the part of the digestive system located at the top of the trachea. This is an unusual diagnosis and condition treated by gastroenterologists. It is also an uncommon cancer associated with chronic reflux.

CAUSES.  GERD is certainly a factor in the development of laryngeal carcinoma, even among those who do not smoke or consume alcohol. Tobacco and alcohol, nonetheless, generally make the situation worse. The reasons are that tobacco and alcohol greatly increase the likelihood of GERD by

1.  decreasing LES basal pressure
2.  promoting esophageal dysmotility
3.  reducing mucosal resistance
4.  delaying gastric emptying
5.  stimulating gastric acid secretion[4]

SYMPTOMS.  In addition to the symptoms of GERD discussed in Chapter 3, people with laryngeal cancer may also experience

1.  chronic cough
2.  cervical dysphagia
3.  globus pharyngeus (a feeling that there is a lump in the throat)
4.  chronic laryngitis
5.  laryngeal/tracheal stenosis (a narrowing of the larynx or trachea)[5]

Anyone experiencing any of these symptoms should see a doctor immediately.

## Adenocarcinoma

Adenocarcinoma is a carcinoma (cancer) in which the cells are arranged in the form of glands. White men are four times more likely to develop adenocarcinoma than black men and eight times more likely to develop it than women, black or white. Adenocarcinoma also occurs somewhere between 30 to 40 percent more often in patients with Barrett's esophagus than people in the general population. Between 59 to 86 percent of adenocarcinomas occur in patients with Barrett's esophagus[6]. Approximately half of all esophageal cancers are adenocarcinoma[7].

CAUSES.  As we have discussed earlier, adenocarcinoma is generally the last stage in the progression from GERD to erosive esophagitis to Barrett's esophagus to adenocarcinoma. The primary cause is GERD, which may be complicated by a lack of diagnosis, failure to treat the symptoms of GERD, poor lifestyle choices, failure to take prescribed medications, or lack of conscientious follow-up by a gastroenterologist. The fact is however, that even with appropriate follow-up and surveillance by your doctor, patients may still develop this condition. Adequate medical evaluation and treatment by your doctor however, can minimize this risk.

SYMPTOMS.  Because adenocarcinoma of the esophagus is so often a result of untreated or undiagnosed Barrett's esophagus, patients with adenocarcinoma of the esophagus may experience the symptoms common to those with Barrett's esophagus, including chest pain, heartburn, sour mouth, persistent cough, and throat pain. However, since adenocarcinoma is such a serious disease, patients may additionally experience weight loss, abdominal pain, and dysphagia.

Unfortunately, some patients with even advanced cases of esophageal adenocarcinoma experience few symptoms until they have an advanced, incurable form of the disease. Needless to say, anyone with symptoms of GERD or Barrett's esophagus should be examined by a doctor as soon as possible, particularly if symptoms are severe, or if symptoms are chronic for a specific diagnosis.

DIAGNOSIS. Diagnosis of adenocarcinoma of the esophagus is made by collecting samples of esophaogeal tissue with an endoscope. The tissue samples are sent to a pathologist for a biopsy to determine whether or not the tissue is cancerous.

TREATMENT. The prognosis for patients who receive a diagnosis of adenocarcinoma during a routine endoscopic surveillance is much more favorable than for patients whose disease has progressed to an advanced stage. The prognosis for patients with any type of cancer is better if the diagnosis is made early in the development of cancerous tumors. Therefore, the earlier the condition can be diagnosed, the better. If detected early, and treated with chemotherapy or surgery, survival rates may be as high as 80 percent. Anyone suffering from Barrett's esophagus should seek early diagnosis and regular treatment from a gastroenterologist. The survival rate of patients who are not diagnosed until the disease has reached an advanced stage is approximately 11 percent.

ENDNOTES

1 Spechler SJ. Adenocarcinoma of the gastroesophageal junction. Clinical Perspectives in Gastroenterology. March/April, 1999;96.

2 MP Ritter, S Oberg, TR DeMeester, JH Peters, M Gadenstatter, PF Crookes, M Fein, CG Bremner. University of Southern California, Department of Surgery, Los Angeles, CA. Duodenogastroesophageal reflux in patients with short segment Barrett's esophagus. Abstract DDW The Society for Surgery of the Alimentary Tract, 1997.

3 Cameron AJ and Lomboy CT. Barrett's esophagus: Age, prevalence, and extent of columnar epithelium. Gastroenterology, 1992: 103 (4) 1241-5.

4 Grant, JC, Quinn, FB. Gastroesophageal reflux disease and the otolaryngologic manifestations. Department of Otolaryngology, UTMB, Grand Rounds, February 3, 1999. Available at: www.utmb.edu.otoref/grnds/GERD-9902/GERD-9902.html.

5 Ibid.

6 Brenton L, Harris BA, Kemp H, Kernstine MD. Virtual Hospital, University of Iowa Health Care. Available at: www.vh.org;Providers/Textbooks/EsophagealCarcinoma/06Adenocarcinoma.html

7 Farivar, M. Available at: www.web.GERD.com/Adencarcinoma.htm.

# 17

# SPECIAL CASES

## *Pregnant Women &*
## *Other Populations*

GERD IS OFTEN DIFFICULT TO DIAGNOSE IN adults who have few physical challenges. Diagnosing GERD can be even more difficult in those whose life has undergone a sudden physical change. Pregnancy, serious illness, or disease, an elderly person with other health issues, handicapped individuals, or infants and small children, for example, may have difficulty expressing the discomfort or pain caused by GERD. Here are special cases and how are they treated.

### *Pregnant Women*

Pregnant women are probably the most likely group of people to experience GERD. In fact, it is estimated that more than 80 percent of pregnant women experience heartburn at least some time in their pregnancy. What causes so much GERD in pregnant women?

WEIGHT GAIN. Weight gain in anyone can cause GERD. Weight gain in pregnant women is especially likely to result in discomfort since the weight is nearly all in the mid-section of the body. As the pregnancy progresses, the additional weight exerts increasing pressure on the stomach and other digestive organs.

HORMONAL CHANGES. During pregnancy, the hormonal balance in a woman's body changes dramatically. One side effect of the increase in progesterone is the slowing of digestion. While this slowing of digestion is may allow the mother to absorb as many nutrients as possible, the result is that the food remains in the stomach longer and can cause GERD.

FETAL ACTIVITY. As the baby grows, its activity in the womb becomes decidedly more pronounced. In the final trimester, the rolling and kicking of the fetus often results in sudden pressure on the stomach. If the baby is especially active after the mother has just eaten, episodes of reflux are likely to occur.

NAUSEA. For reasons that are not entirely understood, some pregnant women experience nausea, particularly during the first trimester of their pregnancy. If a woman already has damage to the esophagus, frequent regurgitation can further irritate the esophageal tissue. If she was not subject to reflux prior to her pregnancy, repeated vomiting can begin to corrode the esophageal lining.

Since pregnant women are generally already under a doctor's care when the symptoms of GERD develop, they can be diagnosed easily.

DIAGNOSIS. Since GERD is so common in pregnant women , obstetricians and gynecologists can prescribe appropriate treatment and monitor it effectively throughout the pregnancy. Usually, a pregnant woman is referred to a gastroenterologist only if her symptoms are unusual or severe.

TREATMENT. Some of the drugs used to treat people who are not pregnant are probably also safe for pregnant women, although even nonprescription drugs should not be taken unless approved by a doctor. There is not a lot of evidence that there is any great harm in pregnant women taking drugs like H2 blockers and PPI's. Since it is not ethical to experiment with these drugs on pregnant women, these medications are not generally considered safe and should be used cautiously. A pregnant woman should have her physician review any medications.

It is generally not a good idea for women to take herbal remedies while pregnant because of the lack of hard data in support of many of these remedies. Many herbal remedies contain more than one active ingredient that could be of risk to the developing fetus. If you are considering taking herbs during pregnancy, please consult your physician first to ensure that the supplement is safe. Your physician should be able to tell you if there is adequate data to confirm its safety for use during pregnancy.

Lifestyle changes, such as elevating the head of the bed, eating smaller meals, and avoiding known GERD-causing foods are also often suggested to pregnant women. With all patients, pregnant or not, these changes are generally recommended before prescribing medications anyway. As none of these suggestions would be harmful to your baby, try them first. If GERD persists, then consult your doctor about what medications, if any, might be safe for you.

It is emphatically recommended that pregnant women avoid smoking and alcohol consumption throughout their pregnancy.

## Infants

As every parent knows, particularly first-time parents, it is often difficult to know just what a baby wants. When a baby cries, it can mean that any number of things are wrong—hunger, a wet diaper, an uncomfortable position, boredom, or just the desire to be picked up. In addition, some of the symptoms that point to GERD in an adult— such as spitting up, not sleeping well, or a lot of burping—may be perfectly normal in a baby. How does a gastroenterologist know if a baby has GERD?

In general, what physicians look for are extremes. A little spitting up is normal. A lot of vomiting is not. Likewise, if a baby has a full stomach, a dry diaper, and continues to cry for an extended period, chances are something more serious is wrong. Another clue may be a lot of respiratory problems or clear signs that the baby is in pain, such as arching its back or an inability to sleep. Recurrent asthma or airway problems can mean a lot in a young child. It could be allergy to mites, dust, or a poor environment. It could be asthma or it could be GERD. Since GERD is quite common in infants, this should certainly be considered.

Often the problem, even if it turns out to be GERD, is a temporary one. Although most full-term babies are fully developed, many premature babies are born before all their systems are mature. For example, it is possible that the lower esophageal sphincter (LES) may just not be working quite right yet.

In any case, if your baby exhibits any of the symptoms described above, you should certainly consult your pediatrician and ask whether GERD may be the problem. If the situation is serious enough, your pediatrician may suggest that you consult a pediatric gastroenterologist whose specialty is treating GERD in children. Pediatric gastroenterologists have extensive experience with GERD in children and are the best resources for such questions. Gastroenterologists who treat adults see these patients much less frequently.

As with pregnant women, often the same medications that are used to treat adults are used for infants. Typically, these drugs are prescribed in much smaller dosages. Similarly, lifestyle changes, like propping the head of the baby's crib up, holding the baby upright for a time after eating, or giving the baby more frequent, smaller meals may help control the GERD. If the problem persists, occasionally surgery can help, even in very young infants.

## Children

As with infants, it is sometimes difficult to diagnose GERD in children until they are old enough to clearly indicate what is bothering them. In younger children, GERD may be the problem if the child has symptoms similar to those of infants, such as vomiting, crying, inability to sleep, and pain in the upper chest.

When they take their child to the doctor, parents are asked by the physician to provide the same information asked of an adult—a week's food diary, a week's activity diary, and a list of any medications the child may be taking. In addition, parents are asked to be aware of whether the child has been eating exceptionally large meals, drinking a lot of carbonated beverages or beverages containing caffeine, lying down or going to bed shortly after eating, or experiencing pain or discomfort in the upper chest.

Chocolate, milk, and high-fat foods are a problem for the average child. In fact, most American children eat excessive amounts of fatty foods. Although the vast majority of them can tolerate this type of diet with no problem whatsoever, a subset of children may benefit significantly from dietary changes if they exhibit symptoms of GERD. The challenge is getting a child to change his or her their diet, since children seem to love fatty food. Other symptoms in children with GERD may include a sour taste in the mouth, a persistent cough, or vomiting.

For children, the first course of action is lifestyle change: propping up the head of the bed; eating smaller, more frequent meals; remaining upright at least an hour before going to bed; avoiding vigorous exercise immediately after eating; and cutting down on carbonated drinks and foods that may exacerbate GERD.

If these do not work, medication may be recommended. Fortunately, most of the medications that work for adults also work for children, although they are, of course, given in smaller dosages. In a few instances, surgery may be recommended.

In all cases, however, no medication should be given to a child on a regular basis without a doctor's recommendation. Under no circumstances should adult prescription medication be shared with a child.

## The Elderly

Elderly people, like pregnant women, often experience GERD because of changes in their body chemistry and physiology.

For many elderly people, GERD may have been a long-term problem, but one that has gone untreated, particularly among elderly people who are smokers or who drink a good deal of alcohol. Years of irritation to the esophagus may have eroded the esophageal tissue, occasionally resulting in pre-cancerous conditions like erosive esophagitis, ulcerative esophagitis, or Barrett's esophagus. In more severe cases, the esophagitis may have already become adenocarcinoma.

Elderly people are also more likely to have developed diabetes and other illnesses that can lead to GERD. Or they may have developed a hiatal hernia. These patients, may also experience muscle weakness or neurologic degeneration, have developed difficulties with clearing their secretions, and may be prone to GERD, particularly those who are confined to bed or a wheelchair.

Among some elderly people, arthritis or simply a lack of exercise may have led to a more sedentary lifestyle. Their diet may have changed significantly, particularly those who live alone. They may have become accustomed to going to bed shortly after the evening meal or napping right after lunch.

Multiple ailments may have also led to the consumption of a wide variety of medications, some of them reacting adversely to others. Even though elderly persons may have lost weight or significantly altered activity level, they may have continued to take the same dosages of medications they took when they were younger and more active. When medication has been changed to reflect changes in physiology, because metabolism has slowed, the drugs may act more slowly or remain in the system longer than previously. Any combination of these issues places the elderly at significant risk for reflux.

As with all patients, it is extremely important that elderly people, or people who care for them, provide the doctor with as much information as possible about the person's lifestyle, eating habits, and medications. Omission of just one fact in treating an elderly person can make diagnosis more difficult or result in the prescription of unhelpful medications.

Because GERD behaves pretty much the same in an elderly person's body as it does in that of a child or a younger adult, the treatment of the elderly is also the same. A lifestyle change is the first recommendation. If that doesn't work, medications are prescribed. Surgery may be recommended for an elderly person, but only if the individual is generally in good health.

## People with Serious Diseases

Patients with GERD who have serious diseases may not always benefit from the same treatment as the average patient. For example, a patient with scleroderma, esophageal cancer, or diabetes, for example, is treated quite differently.

In a patient with scleroderma, the underlying problem is a disease that affects the connective tissues of the entire body, in particular, the esophagus. Once the esophagus has become stiff and less pliable, it is less likely to be able to clear secretions, and peristalsis is inhibited. This predisposes the patient to "stasis" (stoppage) of material (food, drink, acid reflux material, for example) in the esophagus, which, in turn, causes poor clearance of the food from the esophagus and allows continued exposure of the epithelial tissue to injury by the acid.

This situation contributes to further inflammation and scarring, eventually making it difficult for the patient to eat. Although acid suppression may help, these patients will find more relief from sitting up (or standing) during meals. Gravity can assist with clearing the esophagus. They may also require pro-motility agents, such as meto-clopramide, to assist in gastric emptying. They may also require surgery even though the prognosis is poor in these patients.

In a patient with esophageal cancer, the mass effect of the tumor on the esophagus will likely impact the normal functioning of the sphincter, making the patient prone to reflux. The tumor may also cause a stricture and narrowing that would ultimately become problematic even if the patient were taking acid-suppressing medicines or if the area were dilated.

In some patients with scleroderma, the mainstay of treatment would actually be chemotherapy, radiation, or surgical excision of the mass. In the absence of these approaches, however, lifestyle changes and eating several small meals a day would be recommended.

In patients with diabetes, the mainstay of treatment would focus upon maintaining strict glucose control, since it has been shown to be the best predictor of improved gastric motility in patients with diabetic gastroparesis (paralysis of the stomach). Once glucose control is achieved, if symptoms persist, then pro-motility agents often help. Again, acid suppression may also help but may not be the primary mode of therapy in these patients.

# 1 8

# COSTS OF GERD
## *Treatment & Insurance Factors*

D EALING WITH THE HEALTHCARE INSURANCE system can be enormously frustrating. There are hundreds of options available and costs vary considerably from one region of the country to another. In general, most healthcare services are more expensive in urban centers and on the coasts than they are in small towns, in the Midwest, and in mountain states, with some exceptions.

While it is not possible to present specific information regarding the costs for treating GERD, the general costs of some medications are included in the following pages. This chapter also offers an overview of how the insurance system works in this country and suggests questions you should ask your doctor as you work together to decide what type of treatment may be the best for you.

### Health Insurance

Most health insurance today is provided as part of an employee's benefits package. People who are self-employed or who work for companies that do not provide health insurance benefits often purchase such insurance through an association or other organization in order to take advantage of group rates. In any case, such insurance is known as private health insurance, because it is not managed by the government. The most common kinds of private health insurance are described below.

Private Health Insurance

Private health insurance provided by employers generally falls into one of three categories: indemnity plans, preferred provided organizations (PPOs), or health maintenance organizations (HMOs).

INDEMNITY PLANS.  If your employer has an indemnity insurance plan, generally that means that you may choose your own physician, hospital, and pharmacy. When you use a service, the physician, hospital, or pharmacy will bill you and/or your employer in one of four ways:

1.  The service provided may submit the bill to your employer (or directly to your employer's insurance carrier) after which the employer pays all of the costs.
2.  The service provider may bill your employer for a portion of the costs and require you to pay the difference.
3.  The service provider may require you to pay the total cost of the service or medication, and then collect reimbursement.
4.  Require that you pay your portion of the bill at the time of your office visit, hospital stay, or prescription purchase and they (the doctor, hospital, or pharmacy) will bill the employer's portion directly to the employer.

PREFERRED PROVIDER ORGANIZATIONS.  Preferred Provider Organizations (PPOs) are groups of physicians (and/or hospitals) that have an agreement with local employers that they will offer discounts on services if the employers agree to use their services exclusively. If your employer has an agreement with a PPO, then you, as an employee, will be given a list of physicians and hospitals from which to choose. When you have an office visit or a hospital stay, the payment procedure will be the same as if you had an indemnity plan (see above). You will often have to pay a small co-payment, usually ranging from $10 to $25 per visit.

HEALTH MAINTENANCE ORGANIZATIONS. Your employer may have an agreement with a Health Maintenance Organization (HMO). HMOs differ from PPOs in that an HMO is often a physical facility with a staff of either primary care providers or primary care providers and specialists. Some HMOs also run hospitals and pharmacies as well. If this is the case, you will be required to use this facility and this staff of doctors. In some cases, you may be able to choose a physician from the HMO staff and you will see that physician for all of your visits. In other cases, a physician will be assigned to you. In yet other instances, when you make an appointment, you may be seen by what-ever doctor is working at the HMO at that time.

Usually an employer will not pay for the cost of visiting a special-ist, such as a gastroenterologist, unless that specialist is on the staff of the HMO or you are referred to the specialist by the primary care physi-cian at the HMO. As with indemnity plans or PPOs, whether you pay a portion of the costs of this service and how you pay it will depend on what kind of arrangement you or your employer has with the HMO. Again, a co-payment is usually charged at the time of service.

GOVERNMENT HEALTH INSURANCE
MEDICARE.   Medicare is a federal healthcare program that was cre-ated in 1965 by the U.S. Department of Heath and Human Services (formerly the Department of Health, Education and Welfare) to help assure that older Americans would have access to affordable health-care. In 1972, the program was expanded to include people with dis-abilities and end-stage renal disease. Medicare is divided into two plans, A and B. Plan A is hospital insurance; Plan B is insurance that covers other costs, such as doctor office visits. If you are over the age of 65 and you and/or your spouse have worked and paid Medicare

taxes for at least 10 years you are eligible to receive Part A at no additional cost to you. (If you and/or your spouse have not worked and paid Medicare taxes for 10 years, you may have to purchase Plan A.)

Plan B is optional and must be purchased. (The current cost is $54 per month.)

Originally Medicare was strictly a reimbursement plan, but now physicians and hospitals can bill Medicare directly. For more specific information about Medicare, visit the official Medicare Web site (www.Medicare.gov).

As with other health insurance plans, not all costs of office visits or hospital stays are covered by Medicare. If you qualify for Medicare, you should ask your doctor what portion of your treatment is covered and what you should expect to pay. In most states, the cost of prescription medications is not covered by Medicare except those medications received during a hospital stay.

In August, 2002, the federal government began an experimental program that offers 11 million Medicare participants in 23 states the option to use PPOs. (It also allows participants to choose physicians outside the PPO network if they agree to pay extra.) Under this plan, for the first time prescription drug coverage will also be offered outside the hospital.

MEDIGAP INSURANCE.  Until August 2002, Medicare had not paid for prescription medications except those used in the hospital or for those who receive 100 percent of all healthcare costs. Many people purchase a Medigap health insurance policy (and will continue to need to do so in those states not included in the experimental plan). While Medigap policies supplement Medicare, they are not affiliated with or regulated by the federal government. There are now many Medigap policies available and they offer different benefits. The cost of Medigap policies varies considerably. Always shop around before purchasing such a policy. The American Association of Retired Persons (AARP) has a lot of good information about Medigap Insurance and will provide that information to you free of charge. You can reach AARP at www.AARP.org., call them at 1-800-424-3410, or write to them at 601 E St. NW, Washington, DC, 20049.

MEDICAID.  Medicare was created to provide older working Americans with affordable healthcare. Medicaid was created to help the indigent. Medicaid is a combination state and federal program, and qualifications vary from state to state. Medicaid generally pays all or at least most of the cost of office visits, hospital stays, and medications, but the regulations involving how that care can be received are generally more stringent that those for Medicare recipients. Usually, to receive Medicaid a person must be indigent enough to qualify for a state's welfare program. To find out if you qualify for Medicaid, you can visit the official Medicaid website (www.cms.hhs.gov) or call the agency in your community that provides Welfare benefits.

HOW HEALTH CARE COSTS ARE DETERMINED.  Theoretically, physicians, hospitals, and pharmaceutical companies can charge what they wish for their services. Since most patients and employers have choices about what they will pay for, most healthcare providers determine prices for products and services based on what Diagnosis Related Group (DRG) the service or procedure falls within. DRGs were created in 1983 to help contain Medicare costs in hospitals. Currently, DRGs are being used by private insurers to determine the "usual and customary" costs of a particular procedure. There are now 503 possible classifications of diagnoses in the DRG listings. Most physicians and hospitals can generally find one that fits the situation faced by a particular patient.

Since the U.S. healthcare system is not controlled by the government, physicians and hospitals are free to charge whatever they want. Most private insurance companies and/or employers as well as federal insurance providers, like Medicare and Medicaid, however, will only pay the costs estimated by the DRGs.

## Medical Tests

Like office visits and hospital stays, the costs of medical tests are generally determined by what DRG they fall within. These costs, like the costs of other services, may vary by geographical location or whether the tests are performed in a large city. Thanks to computer technology, many diagnostic tests can now be performed right in the doctor's office and results given to the patient within a few minutes. Other diagnostic tests are performed either at an independent laboratory or testing facility. Like other medical services, the private insurer, Medicare, or Medicaid may require that tests be performed at a specific location by a specific provider. Before you have a diagnostic test performed, you should ask both your doctor and your insurance carrier what the cost of such a test will be and where it may be performed. Only then can you determine what the cost to you will be.

## Surgery

A system has also been created to help standardize the costs of surgical procedures. Although diagnostic coding was done as early as the 17th century in England, it wasn't until the late 1940s that the World Health Organization published the International Classification (IC) of Diseases. In 1988, a provision of the Medicare Catastrophic Coverage Act required that each Medicare Part B claim include the appropriate IC codes. Now most insurers insist on the inclusion of these codes, as well, when determining how much they will reimburse physicians for medical services including surgery. Still, it is often very difficult to estimate the exact cost of a particular surgery. Often, only until the surgery is underway will the surgeon know for sure the extent of the costs. Before you have any service provided, it is a good idea to talk to both your insurance provider and your doctor to determine what the anticipated costs may be.

## *Medications*

Most private healthcare plans, Medicaid (and now in some states, Medicare) cover at least a portion of the cost of prescription medications. Very few insurance plans cover the cost of over-the-counter (nonprescription) medications. Whether you have an indemnity plan, a PPO plan, or are part of an HMO, your employer (or some Medicare plans or Medicaid) will cover the costs of your medicines in one of several ways:

1. Cover the cost of all of your medications. (Few companies do this.)
2. Cover the total cost of some of your medications. (For example, if you work for a pharmaceutical company, the company may cover the total cost of all medications they manufacture and give you a discount on medications they don't manufacture.)
3. Charge you a fixed fee for every prescription (e.g., $10) no matter what it is.
4. Share the cost of medications with you through a co-pay arrangement in which you pay a certain percentage or dollar amount for your medications.

OBTAINING MEDICATION. You should be aware that most HMOs and PPOs often restrict physicians' choice of medicines they can prescribe to you. In GERD, for example, there may be five PPIs, all similar in action and effect, of which your insurance company may only allow you to choose one. In addition, your insurer may also restrict the number of tablets your physician will be allowed to prescribe per day or month.

Therefore, if you have particularly serious GERD that responds only to twice a day therapy and your insurer thinks that you should be taking only one tablet a day, the doctor will not be able to prescribe the twice a day dose because the pharmacy will not fill the prescription.

This situation typically results in a lot of paperwork and time spent by your physician (and often by you) to fight for the medicine and the dose that your physician feels you need. For this reason, some doctors are actually pulling themselves out of HMOs to avoid such time-consuming efforts and administrative hassles. Many doctors argue that this is time that would be better spent with the patient.

When choosing your insurance coverage, keep the prescription drug plan rules in mind, particularly if you have a known underlying aliment that will require on-going prescription medicine.

If you are part of an indemnity plan, your employer may require that you get all your medications (at least the medications they are paying for or paying some of the cost of) at a specific pharmacy. In some cases, the employer may require that you order your prescription medications from a mail order or internet-based pharmacy.

BRAND NAMES VS. GENERICS.  Some medications (such as Nexium) have no generic equivalents because the pharmaceutical company that developed the medication still holds the patent to the medication. The patent has now expired on other medications (like Axid, Zantac and Pepcid) and generic versions of these medications are now available. While there is some on-going debate about whether the generic versions of medications are as effective as the originals because they are pharmacologically similar, the end effect should be about the same. Some employers only pay for the generic medication.

Regulations about generic medications also vary from state to state. In some states the law requires that a pharmacist offer you the option of purchasing the generic version of the medication. In other states, the pharmacist may simply substitute the generic version of the medication for what the physician prescribed and not tell the patient. In yet other states, the pharmacist may even substitute an entirely different medication from the one your doctor prescribed.

Before you have a prescription filled, you should check with your doctor to see what the law is in your state and whether or not your doctor feels you should have the brand name medication or whether a generic will work just as well.

AVERAGE COSTS OF **GERD** MEDICATIONS. The costs of all medications can vary greatly depending on where you buy your medications, how they are purchased, what dosage you take and how your insurer reimburses you. To give you a general idea of the cost of GERD medications, the following chart reflects what each medication would cost if you paid full price for it at a Midwestern chain grocery store pharmacy in early 2003.

| PRESCRIPTION MEDICATION | FORM | DOSAGE | QUANTITY | FULL COST |
|---|---|---|---|---|
| Asiphex | Tablets | 20 mg | 30 | $129.99 |
| Axid | Tablets | 150 mg | 30 | $185.19 |
| Generic Axid | Tablets | 150 mg | 30 | $53.79 |
| Nexium | Tablets | 40 mg | 30 | $134.39 |
| Nexium | Tablets | 20 mg | 30 | $134.39 |
| Pepcid | Tablets | 20 mg | 60 | $123.39 |
| Generic Pepcid | Tablets | 20 mg | 60 | $16.75 |
| Prevacid | Tablets | 30 mg | 30 | $137.89 |
| Prilosec | Tablets | 20 mg | 30 | $140.19 |
| Protonix | Tablets | 20 mg | 30 | $103.09 |
| Reglan | Tablets | 10 mg | 30 | $117.49 |
| Generic Reglan | Tablets | 10 mg | 30 | $59.59 |
| Tagamet | Tablets | 300 mg | 60 | $71.19 |
| Generic Tagamet | Tablets | 300 mg | 60 | $19.59 |
| Zantac | Tablets | 150 mg | 60 | $118.19 |
| Generic Zantac | Tablets | 150 mg | 60 | $10.80 |

| Non-prescription Medication | Form | Dosage | Quantity | Full Cost |
|---|---|---|---|---|
| Alka Setlzer Heartburn Relief | Tablets | 2 tabs as needed | 30 | $3.95 |
| Axid AR | Tablets | 1 tab before a meal | 30 | $9.59 |
| Gaviscon | Tablets | 2 tabs 4 x /day | 100 | $8.99 |
| Store brand Gaviscon | Tablets | 2 tabs 4 x /day | 100 | $5.69 |
| Maalox | Liquid | 2-4 tsp., 4 x /day | 12 fl. oz. | $4.25 |
| Store brand Maalox | Liquid | 2-4 tsp. 4 x /day | 12 fl. oz. | $3.19 |
| Mylanta | Gelcaps | 2-4 gelcaps, 4 x /day | 24 | $3.59 |
| Mylanta | Liquid | 2-4 tsp. between meals and at bedtime | 12 fl. oz. | $4.75 |
| Store brand Mylanta | Liquid | 2-4 tsp. between meals and at bedtime | 12 fl. oz. | $3.55 |
| Pepcid AC | Tablets | 1 tab 2 x /day | 30 | $23.99 |
| Store brand Pepcid | Tablets | 1 tab 2 x /day | 90 | $12.99 |
| Phillips Milk of Magnesia | Liquid | 1-3 tsp. 4 x /day | 12 fl. oz. | $5.19 |
| Store brand Phillips Milk of Magnesia | Liquid | 1-3 tsp. 4 x /day | 12 fl. oz. | $3.69 |
| Rolaids | Lozenge | 1-4 hourly | 150 | $4.49 |
| Tagamet HB | Tablets | 2 tabs in 24 hours | 30 | $9.39 |
| Store brand Tagamet | Tablets | 2 tabs in 24 hours | 30 | $6.85 |
| Tums | Tablets | 2-3 tabs as symptoms occur | 150 | $4.49 |
| Store brand Tums | Tablets | 2-3 tabs as symptoms occur | 116 | $2.99 |
| Zantac 75 | Tablets | 2 tabs in 24 hours | 105 | $21.49 |
| Store brand Zantac | Tablets | 2 tabs in 24 hours | 60 | $11.15 |

tab=tablet
tsp.=teaspoons
Tbsp.=tablespoons

The American Association of Retired Persons (AARP) has produced a pamphlet "Drug Smart" that offers suggestions on the various ways prescriptions may be filled and a guide to obtaining the best value for your prescription dollars. To obtain this pamphlet, you may call 1-800-424-3410, write to AARP at 601 E St. NW, Washington, D.C. or visit www.modernmaturity.org. Additional price comparisons may be made by checking with on-line pharmacies.

# 19

## FUTURE TRENDS

### *Endoscopic Procedural Therapies & More*

Many of the therapies used to treat GERD are centuries old. Others are so new they're not yet available outside clinical trials. As discussed in earlier chapters, most people find relief from GERD by altering their diets and/or lifestyles. When those changes do not provide adequate relief, one or more of the medications discussed in Chapter 10 often eliminate the symptoms and help keep the disease under control. When medication is not effective, one or more of the surgeries discussed in Chapter 13 should be considered.

The following endoscopic techniques are also currently available as options to surgery.

### Bard Endoscopic Suturing System

In April 2000, the Bard endoscopic suturing system became available to treat GERD and to improve the function of the weakened or non-functioning LES. During the procedure the surgeon inserts an endoscope through the patient's mouth and into his or her stomach. A device on the end of the endoscope captures a small amount of stomach tissue into which is stitch is made. Several such stitches are then sewn together to create pleats in the wall of the stomach just below the esophagus. This procedure requires no intravenous or topical anesthetic and a topical spray can be used to lessen gagging, but most patients opt for an intravenous anesthetic. The procedure is performed on an outpatient basis, takes about an hour, and seems to have minimal side effects. Patients go home the same day and recover within a few hours.

Unlike many of the other types of surgery, the procedure can be reversed because sutures are used. This is important because some patients need to have the repair tightened or loosened. Since it is a new procedure, no one yet knows how long the repair will last.

## Stretta System

The Stretta system is similar to the Bard endoscopic suturing system in that an endoscope is used and no general anesthesia is required. But instead of stitches, the Stretta system relies on electrodes. Once the endoscope is in place, electrodes burn spots on the muscle that controls the faulty valve, causing flexible scar tissue to form. It is still not known whether the scar tissue actually strengthens the valve or whether the heat generated by the electrodes repairs the nerves that caused the LES to malfunction.

There is still some controversy surrounding the use of this procedure because it is permanent and the long-term effects are still unknown. It has recently been approved for use in patients with refractory reflux (reflux that does not readily respond to treatment) who do not wish to have either anti-reflux suturing or surgical therapy.

## Enteryx Therapy

Enteryx therapy was approved by the FDA on April 22, 2003 to treat acid reflux. During the procedure, a permanent, implantable biopolymer (consisting of a liquid solution containing a polymer and a solvent) is injected with a tiny needle into the lower esophageal sphincter just above the entrance into the stomach. Once injected, the solution solidifies into a spongelike material. This therapy augments the lower esophageal sphincter by reinforcing it to enhance the barrier to reflux. The procedure can be done on an outpatient basis and takes about one hour to perform. A one-year study found that up to 70 percent of patients who had undergone Enteryx therapy were able to eliminate their dependency on daily medicines. However, the safety of this therapy beyond one year of treatment has not been established. Retrosternal pain (pain behind the sternum), dysphagia, and fever have been seen in some patients after such therapy. This therapy is not approved for all patients and a thorough discussion of its potential use is necessary for all patients considering it.

## Dilation of the Esophagus

Of course, not all problems related to GERD involve the LES. Some surgeries, instead of treating the cause of GERD, are designed to repair the resulting damage. One of these problems is stricture of the esophagus. This condition occurs when reflux has been allowed to occur often and long enough that scar tissue (strictures) has formed on the lining of the esophagus. This scar tissue has narrowed the esophagus to the point that swallowing may be difficult. For patients with these strictures, medication, diet, and lifestyle changes won't help. And the problem won't go away on its own. Endoscopic intervention in the form of dilation is generally required.

In this procedure, the esophagus is enlarged by a water-filled rubber bag or a metal rod called a bougie. While this procedure is generally safe, there is a slight risk that a perforation of the esophagus could occur. This would be a very serious situation requiring immediate emergency care. But this rarely happens, particularly if the gastroen-terologist is experienced in performing this procedure.

While effective, this procedure does not always provide a long-term solution and may have to be repeated every few months. Per-sistent scars may have to be surgically removed.

Still, endoscopic dilation is always the first choice of therapy for stricture of the esophagus. It is performed on an outpatient basis and is tolerated much better than surgery by most patients.

## Future Trends

Although more is known about GERD than ever before, the search for therapies that are more effective, easier to administer, and more afford-able continues. Several such therapies are now in experimental stages.

EXPERIMENTAL MEDICATION: CELEBREX (CELECOXIB)  This anti-inflammatory medication, used primarily for treatment of arthritis, is now being tried on an experimental basis for treatment of Barrett's esophagus. The hope is that Celebrex will be successful in regressing the development of the pre-cancerous tissue typically found in those who suffer from this disease[1].

EXPERIMENTAL SURGERIES.  Beginning in the 1950s with Dr. Nis-sen's fundloplication, a variety of surgical techniques have been used to reshape the LES (lower esophageal sphincter) and prevent acid reflux. Although the procedure was made minimally invasive in the 1990s, it did not always provide the desired result.

Now under experimentation is a surgical procedure in which in which plexiglas microspheres, (polymethylmethacrylate beads), now used to treat skin defects and wrinkles, are implanted in esophageal sphincters. These implants increase the thickness of the LES folds and, hopefully, will decrease the incidence of acid reflux[2].

Another experimental surgery is the gatekeeper reflux repair system. This experimental device consists of an expandable hydrogel prosthesis that can be implanted into the wall of the esophagus by the use of an endoscope. It is a minimally invasive procedure, performed on an outpatient basis and, so far, appears to cause no permanent damage to the esophagus. The prostheses are made of the same material as contact lenses and are about the same diameter as a pencil lead. When inserted into the esophageal wall, they act as barriers to acid reflux without blocking food from entering the stomach[3].

The endoscopic mucosal resection is another experimental treatment for those suffering from Barrett's esophagus. In this procedure, an instrument lifts the esophageal lining and injects a solution under it or applies suction to it and then cuts it off, much in the same way colon polyps are removed. The diseased lining that has been removed is then sent to a laboratory, which analyzes it for malignancy. This procedure cannot be used to remove large sections of lining, but seems to have promise in removing small cancers or localized areas of high-grade dysphasia[4].

EXPERIMENTAL THERAPIES.    Because Barrett's esophagus is such a serious side effect of GERD, several therapies are now undergoing experimental trials with the hope of finding a way to prevent the lining of the esophagus from producing pre-cancerous cells.

Photodynamic therapy (PDT) consists of giving the patient a light-sensitizing drug (a photosensitizer) through a vein or by mouth. This drug sensitizes all the cells in the body— including the Barrett's esophagus cells—to light. The photosensitizing drug tends to concentrate in precancerous or cancerous cells. A laser is then inserted into the esophagus and its light activates the photosensitizing agent, destroying the Barrett's lining. After treatment the cells are sloughed off. The patients are then given strong antacids to prevent reflux while healthy esophageal cells grow back. PDT is also being tested for use in the lungs, on the skin, head, and neck.

At this time, the therapy can have severe side effects, including nausea, esophageal scarring, and sunburn, if any skin on the body is exposed to sunlight for up to six weeks following the procedure[5].

Another experimental therapy, thermal ablation, works like photodynamic therapy. It destroys the precancerous cells in the esophagus. The difference is that thermal ablation uses heat instead of light. Three thermal ablation techniques are now in the experimental stage: multipolar polar electrocautery, argon plasma coagulation (APC), and laser ablation (KTP).

In multipolar polar electrocautery, an electric wire is inserted into the esophagus and the dysplasia is literally burned away. In argon plasma coagulation, a stream of argon gas is released into the esophagus along with an electric current that burns away the dysplasia. In laser ablation, lasers are aimed at the precancerous cells, destoying them[6].

CRYOTHERAPHY AND ULTRASONIC THERAPY. Two other experimental therapies are now being considered. Cyrotherapy would use liquid nitrogen to freeze the diseased epithelial cells. Ultrasonic therapy would use sound waves to destroy the diseased cells. Both of these therapies have been used in animal experiments but have not been tested on humans.

FOOTNOTES
1 National Cancer Institute Press Release, February 27, 2001.
2 Mayo Clinic Jacksonville, www.mayo.edu/mcj/gastro/esophcancer.html).
3 University of Kentucky press release, August 9, 2002.
4 www.barrettsinfo.com/content/9_investigational-therapies.htm
5 Winthrop University Hospital Press Release, June 26, 2000.
6 Mayo Clinic Jacksonville, www.mayo.edu/mcj/gastro/esophacancer.html

# 20

# RECIPES FOR GERD
# PATIENTS
*Healthful, Delicious Choices*

P REPARED BY HEATHER HEDRICK, ASSISTANT director of the Center for Educational Services, National Institute for Fitness and Sport. Heather is a registered dietician and also a world-class triathlete.

The key to proper nutrition for everyone, but especially those suffering from GERD, is balance, variety, and moderation. You should keep these basic principles in mind with each meal and snack you consume throughout the day. An easy rule of thumb in preparing a healthy meal is to aim for three different foods and, as we suggested in the chapter on healthy eating, to eat slowly enough to enjoy them all.

A good diet for a GERD sufferer has some limitations that we have discussed in previous chapters. But fortunately for you, a GERD-healthy diet is not as restrictive as diets people with other types of gastrointestinal problems must follow. In the United States, we have a huge variety of foods available so the only limitation to an interesting and healthy diet is your own creativity.

Following On the following pages are some suggestions to get you started:

## *Breakfast*

### MIXED GRAIN HOT CEREAL
Makes 2 servings

*This cereal contains a combination of soluble and insoluble fiber from the oatmeal and bulgur wheat, respectively. It really warms the body on a cold winter morning! You can substitute other whole grains such as quinoa, kamut, or millet for the oatmeal or bulgur wheat. For an interesting alternative, substitute 1/4 cup cooked or canned pumpkin for the bulgur wheat.*

### Ingredients
1/2 cup oatmeal
1/2 cup bulgur wheat

1 cup milk or soy milk
1/2 cup raisins
brown sugar, to taste

### Directions
In a medium saucepan set over medium-high heat, boil 2 cups water. Add the oatmeal and bulgur wheat. Cook for 10 to 15 minutes, stirring occasionally. Divide cereal between two bowls. Top each with 1/2 cup milk, 1/4 cup raisins, and a sprinkling of brown sugar. For further variety, top oatmeal with chopped pecans, sunflower seeds, bananas, or fresh berries.

*Food Groups: grains, dairy/dairy alternative, fruit*

## GET-UP-AND-GO SMOOTHIE
*Makes 1 serving*

*This breakfast can be made in 5 minutes or less. To freeze bananas, allow them to become slightly brown, peel and place in a freezer bag, and freeze overnight. When you prepare your smoothie, take one banana out of the freezer bag and put it directly into the blender with the other ingredients. Combine the smoothie with a piece of toast topped with 1 tablespoon peanut butter, and breakfast is complete!*

### Ingredients
1 banana, frozen
1/2 cup fresh or frozen strawberries
1 cup milk or soy milk
1/2 cup vanilla yogurt
ice (optional)

### Directions
Mix all ingredients in a blender until smooth. Add ice for a thicker shake.

*Food Groups: fruit, dairy/dairy alternative, grain, meat/meat alternative*

BLOOMING-WITH-NUTRITION BLUEBERRY MUFFINS
*Makes 12 muffins*

*Blueberries are filled with antioxidants, which keep our bodies healthy. Whole wheat flour boosts the fiber content slightly. Two egg whites are used instead of a whole egg to decrease the cholesterol. Pecans may be added to the muffin batter for a unique flavor and the benefit of unsaturated fats.*

**Ingredients**
1 cup all-purpose flour
1 cup whole wheat flour
3 teaspoons baking powder
1/2 teaspoon salt
1/3 cup butter or margarine
2/3 cup granulated sugar
2 egg whites
3/4 cup skim milk or soy milk
1 cup fresh or frozen blueberries (if frozen, do not thaw)
1/2 to 1 cup chopped pecans

**Directions**
Preheat oven to 425°F. In a medium bowl, sift flours, baking powder, and salt. In a large bowl, cream the margarine, add sugar, and blend thoroughly. Add egg whites and beat well. Add the flour mixture to the margarine mixture alternately with the milk in three portions. Divide batter into greased muffin tins. Fold in the blueberries and the nuts. Bake 15 to 20 minutes or until golden brown.

*Food Groups: grains, fruit, dairy/dairy alternative*
*Meal Suggestion: One muffin, a fruit salad and a glass of milk*

## Nutty French Toast

*Makes 4 servings*

### Ingredients
3 egg whites
1/2 cup skim milk or soy milk
2 tablespoons creamy peanut butter
1 teaspoon ground cinnamon
1/4 teaspoon ground nutmeg
1 teaspoon honey
non-stick cooking spray
4 slices whole wheat bread
Non-stick cooking spray
1/2 C cup unsweetened applesauce
maple syrup

### Directions
In a small bowl, whisk together the egg whites, milk, peanut butter, spices, and honey until smooth. Coat a frying pan with non-stick cooking spray and set over medium heat. Dip one slice of bread at a time into the egg white mixture, covering both sides, and then place in the pan. Cook each side of the bread 3 minutes or until golden brown. Serve topped with applesauce and syrup. Whole fruit can be used in place of the applesauce.

*Food Groups: grains, fruit, dairy/dairy alternative*
*Meal Suggestion: Nutty French Toast topped with fruit or applesauce, 1 cup skim or soy milk or yogurt*

## Lunch

### HOMEMADE HUMMUS
*Makes 6 servings*

*Store-bought hummus can be high in calories and/or fat if one of the main ingredients is olive oil. This recipe uses the liquid that is packed with the canned beans to give the spread flavor and moistness. Hummus will last about one week in the refrigerator. It is delicious in a sandwich, as a vegetable dip, or as an appetizer spread on crackers.*

### Ingredients
15-ounce can garbanzo beans, with 1/2 tablespoon of the liquid from the can.
1/2 tablespoon lemon juice
2 teaspoons tahini
2 teaspoons ground cumin
2 teaspoons ground coriander
1/2 teaspoon ground black pepper

### Directions
Combine all ingredients in a food processor and blend until smooth. Spread on whole wheat or pita bread with lots of lettuce and tomato.

*Food Groups: grains, fruit, dairy/dairy alternative, meat/meat alternative
Meal Suggestion: Homemade Hummus sandwich on whole wheat bread, 8 ounces low-fat yogurt, 1 piece of whole fruit*

## MIXED BEAN SALAD
*Makes 8 servings*

### Ingredients
15-ounce can kidney beans
15-ounce can black beans
15-ounce can garbanzo beans
1/3 pound radishes, chopped
1/4 cup balsamic vinegar
1 tablespoon Dijon mustard
1/4 cup olive oil
2 teaspoons ground pepper

4 tablespoons parsley
romaine lettuce or spinach leaves

### Directions
In a large bowl, combine the kidney beans, black beans, garbanzo beans, and radishes. Stir to combine. In a small bowl, whisk together the vinegar, mustard, oil, and ground pepper and stir into the bean mixture. Refrigerate until well chilled; serve on a bed of Romaine lettuce or spinach leaves.

*Food Groups: vegetables, meat/meat alternative, grains*
*Meal Suggestion: Mixed Bean Salad on a bed of greens and a bran muffin*

## SPLIT PEA AND HAM SOUP

*Makes 6 to 8 servings*

### Ingredients

1 pound green split peas
1 1/2 cups diced parsnips
1 cup diced cooked ham
1 cup diced carrots
3 teaspoons celery flakes
2 teaspoons dried rosemary
2 teaspoons ground black pepper
1 cup skim or soy milk

### Directions

In a Dutch oven or 3- to 4-quart saucepan, combine the split peas, parsnips, carrots, and spices. Add 7 cups water. Bring mixture to boil over high heat. Reduce heat to low and simmer, covered, for 2 hours, stirring occasionally, or until thick and the water has been absorbed. Stir in the milk. Add the ham and simmer for 5 to 10 minutes, until heated through. If you prefer a smoother texture, before adding the ham, puree the soup in small batches in a blender or food processor. Return blended soup to the saucepan and heat through before serving. (For vegetarian soup, simply eliminate the ham.)

*Food Groups: grains, fruit, meat/meat alternative*
*Meal Suggestion: Split Pea and Ham Soup, tossed salad, and whole grain crackers*

## Asparagus Salad

*Makes 4 servings*

### Ingredients

1 bunch asparagus
1/2 small head of red cabbage
2 tablespoons olive oil
2 to 3 tablespoons balsamic vinegar
gorgonzola cheese (optional)

### Directions

Steam asparagus until just tender. Remove from heat and let cool. Cut asparagus into 1- to 2-inch pieces and place in a medium bowl. Chop cabbage; add to asparagus. Toss oil and vinegar with asparagus and cabbage just before serving.

*Food Groups: vegetables, grains, meat/meat alternative, dairy/dairy alternative*
*Meal Suggestion: Asparagus Salad, 1/2 turkey sandwich on whole wheat bread, glass of skim or soy milk*

## Dinner

### Monkey Bread
*Makes 1 loaf*

#### Ingredients
1/3 cup margarine
1/2 cup sugar
4 egg whites
1 cup all-purpose flour
3/4 cup whole wheat flour
1 teaspoon baking powder
1 teaspoon baking soda
1/2 teaspoon salt
1 teaspoon ground cinnamon
1/4 teaspoon ground nutmeg
1 cup mashed ripe bananas
1/2 cup chopped walnuts or pecans

#### Directions
Preheat oven to 350°F. In a medium bowl cream together the margarine and sugar. Add the egg whites; beat well. In a small bowl, sift together the flours, baking powder, baking soda, salt, cinnamon, and nutmeg. Add to creamed ingredients, alternating with banana, and blending well after each addition. Stir in nuts. Pour into a well-greased 9-x5-x3-inch loaf pan. Bake for 45 to 50 minutes, or until a toothpick inserted in the center of the bread comes out clean.

*Food Groups: grains*

## CHICKEN PESTO PASTA
*Makes 4 servings*

*Most pestos are high in fat because of the amount of oil. This is a lower fat alternative. For a delicious variation, replace some of the basil with fresh broccoli. Broccoli pesto is a great alternative to tomato sauce for pasta dishes.*

## Ingredients
*For Basil Pesto*
2 large cloves garlic, diced
1/4 cup fresh basil
6 tablespoons low-fat yogurt

*For Broccoli Pesto*
3 cups broccoli florets, steamed until just tender
1/4 cup dried basil
1/2 teaspoon black pepper
1/3 cup vegetable broth
1 to 2 tablespoons lemon juice
1 to 2 tablespoons olive oil
2 large cloves garlic

*For the Pasta and Chicken*
4 2two-ounce servings pasta (spaghetti, linguini or fettuccini), cooked and drained
1/4 cup vegetable oil
4 skinless, boneless chicken breasts, cut in bite-size pieces
1 cup fresh mushrooms, sliced
2 tablespoons Parmesan cheese
chopped fresh basil, for garnish

**Directions**

Place all ingredients for either the basil or broccoli pesto in a blender or food processor and blend until mixed well. Set aside. Bring a large pot of water to a boil and prepare pasta according to package directions. While the pasta is boiling, in a large skillet, heat the vegetable oil until hot, but not smoking. Add the chicken and sauté until well done and browned on the outside. During the last 2 or 3 minutes the chicken is cooking, stir in the onion and mushrooms and cook until just tender. Drain the pasta; transfer to a serving bowl. Add the chicken and vegetables and stir in the pesto. Divide pasta evenly among 4 serving plates and sprinkle each with grated Parmesan cheese and chopped basil.

*Food Groups: meat/meat substitute, grains, vegetables, dairy*
*Meal Suggestion: Goes well with a large tossed salad. For a vegetarian meal, eliminate the chicken or replace it with tofu*

## MARINATED TEMPEH WITH VEGETABLES OVER COUSCOUS
*Makes 2 servings*

*Tempeh is a fermented soy product made from whole soybeans. Tempeh has a firmer texture than tofu and a smoky flavor. Tempeh can be found in the refrigerated or freezer section of the grocery store. If you cannot find tempeh in your grocery, substitute firm tofu.*

### Ingredients
1 tablespoon sesame oil
1/4 cup tamari or soy sauce
1/4 cup balsamic vinegar
2 to 3 cloves garlic
1/2 teaspoon curry powder
1/2 teaspoon dried dill
1/4 teaspoon ground ginger
1/4 teaspoon ground cumin
1 package tempeh, cut into cubes
non-stick cooking spray
1 head broccoli, chopped
2 carrots, sliced
2 cups mushrooms
1/2 cup couscous

### Directions
In a large bowl, mix together the sesame oil, tamari or soy sauce, vinegar, garlic, curry powder, dill, ginger, cumin, and tempeh. Cover and refrigerate for 30 minutes.

Meanwhile, prepare the vegetables. Wash the broccoli, carrots, and mushrooms thoroughly; cut into medium-size pieces. In a medium saucepan set over medium heat, bring 3/4 to 1 cup water to a boil. Add couscous, cover, and simmer for 5 minutes. Remove from heat and let stand, covered, for 10 minutes.

Meanwhile, coat a large skillet with non-stick cooking spray; set over medium heat. Saute the vegetables for 5 minutes. Add marinated tempeh, cover, and cook for an additional 5 to 10 minutes, until the tempeh is heated through. Serve the tempeh and vegetables over couscous.

*Food Groups: meat/meat alternative, vegetables, grains, dairy/dairy alternative*
*Meal Suggestion: Marinated Tempeh with Vegetables over Couscous with a glass of skim/soy milk*

## SOUTH OF THE BORDER BURRITOS
*Makes 4 servings*

*This is a great dish to make on the weekend and have as leftovers during the week. The bean and vegetable mix keeps well for two to three days in the refrigerator and can be reheated for a quick and easy dinner. If you are planning to have leftovers, make only the number of burritos to be eaten in the meal and reserve the remaining bean mixture in a container to bake another day.*

### Ingredients
1 tablespoon olive oil
2 medium parsnips
1 yellow pepper, chopped
1/2 tablespoon chili powder (optional)
2 cloves garlic
1 tablespoon oregano
1 teaspoon ground cumin
1 cup canned corn
1 large sweet potato, baked, cooled and diced
1 can black beans or 2 cups cooked, cubed chicken breast
1 tablespoon lime juice (optional)
4 whole wheat tortillas
shredded Monterey Jack or soy cheese (optional)
reduced fat sour cream

### Directions
Preheat oven to 350°F. In a Dutch oven set over medium heat, heat the oil. Add parsnips and yellow pepper and cook, stirring often, 5 to 10 minutes or until soft. Add chili powder, garlic, oregano, and cumin; stir 1 minute. Remove from the heat and stir in corn, sweet potato, beans or chicken, and lime juice. Spoon 1/4

of the bean mixture into each tortilla; add 1 to 2 tablespoons shredded cheese. Roll up each tortilla and place on a greased baking dish, seam side down. Cover with foil; bake 30 minutes. Top with sour cream before serving.

*Food Groups included: meat/meat alternative, vegetables, grains, fruit*
*Meal Suggestion: One burrito, green salad with fresh sliced avocado or a cold tropical fruit salad (mange, papaya, pineapple)*

### GRILLED TUNA STEAKS WITH MANGO SALSA
*Makes 4 servings*

### Ingredients
4 tuna steaks, 4 to 6 ounces each
1 medium mango, peeled and cubed
1/2 cup canned peaches, diced
1/2 cup pineapple chunks, coarsely chopped
1 to 2 tablespoons fresh cilantro, chopped
2 teaspoons white wine vinegar
1 to 2 teaspoons lime juice
3/4 teaspoon ground cumin

### Directions
Preheat broiler or grill. In a medium bowl, combine the mango, peaches, pineapple chunks, cilantro, vinegar, lime juice, and cumin. Refrigerate until ready to use.

Place steaks on a broiler or grill rack sprayed with cooking spray. Cook each side for 4 to 5 minutes or until cooked to desired degree of doneness. Serve tuna with mango salsa.

*Food Groups include: meat/meat alternative, fruit, vegetables*
*Meal Suggestion: Tuna steak and mango salsa and asparagus salad (see lunch recipes)*

## Desserts

### YOGURT AND FRESH FRUIT
*Makes 4 servings*

#### Ingredients
4 cups French vanilla yogurt
Fresh fruit, such as peaches, raspberries, strawberries, or bananas
Toppings, such as crushed peanuts, shaved chocolate, or granola

#### Directions
In a medium bowl, combine the yogurt with the fruit; mix well. Divide among 4 serving bowls and add topping to each. If you are having a party, prepare the fruit and yogurt in bowls, serve your guests, then pass several toppings and let them "mix and match."

*Food Groups: fruit*
*Meal Suggestion: Yogurt and Fresh Fruit makes a cool end to a hot summer or winter meal, and has many fewer calories than ice cream. If fresh fruit is not available, you may substitute canned or frozen fruit, but make sure that you thaw frozen fruit thoroughly and drain both frozen and canned fruit so that your desert is not runny. If you need to lose weight, choose low-fat or fat free yogurt*

# RESOURCES

## Other Books about GERD

Baird, Pat, M.S., R.D., *Be Good to Your Gut: Recipes and Tips for People with Digestive Problems*, Blackwell Science, Inc., Maple–Vail, Binghamton, NY, 1996.

Balch, Dr. James F. and Dr. Morton Walker, *Heartburn and What to Do About It*, Avery Publishing Company, Garden City Park, NY, 1998

Gitnick, Gary, M.D. with Karen Cooksey, *Freedom from Digestive Distress, Medicine Free Relief from Heartburn, Gas, Gloating and Irritable Bowel Syndrome*, Three Rivers Press, New York, 2000.

Harvard Medical School, *The Sensitive Gut*, Fireside, New York, 2001.

Minocha, Anil, M.D. and Christine Adamec, *How to Stop Heartburn: Simple Ways to Heal Heartburn and Acid Reflux*, John Wiley & Sons, Inc., New York, 2001.

Murray, Michael T., ND, *Stomach Aliments and Digestive Disturbances*, Prima Publishing, Rocklin, CA, 1997

Rosenthal, M. Sara, *The Gastro-intestinal Sourcebook*, Lowell House, Lincolnwood, IL, 1997.

*The Sensitive Gut*, Harvard Medical School, New York, NY, 2001

Utley, David S, MD, *Stop the Heartburn*, Lagado Publishing, Woodside, CA, 1996

Wolfe, M. Michael, MD and Thomas Nesi, *The Fire Inside: Extinguishing Heartburn and Related Symptoms*, WW Norton Company, New York, 1996

## ORGANIZATIONS

### AMERICAN ACADEMY OF FAMILY PHYSICIANS
The American Academy of Family Physicians is a national medical organization representing more than 94,000 family physicians, family practice residents and medical students. Founded in 1947, its mission is to preserve and promote the science and art of family medicine and to ensure high quality, cost-effective health care for patients of all ages. Its website provides general information about GERD, as well as other gastrointestinal conditions.
www.familydoctor.org

### AMERICAN COLLEGE OF GASTROENTEROLOGY
The American College of Gastroenterology was founded in 1932 to advance the scientific study and practice of diseases of the gastrointestinal tract. Through the American Journal of Gastroenterology and seminars, the ACG provides its 8,000 members with information and training in the treatment of gastrointestinal diseases. Its website provides both general and very specific information about GERD and other gastrointestinal conditions.
4900 B South 31st Street
Arlington, VA  22206
(703) 820-7400
www.acg.gi.org/patientinfo/frame-gerd.html

### AMERICAN GASTROENTEROLOGICAL ASSOCIATION
The American Gastroenterological Association was founded in 1897 and is the oldest non-profit specialty medical society in the country. Membership consists of approximately 12,000 gastroenterologic physicians and scientists worldwide. The Association publishes *Gastroenterology*, a monthly scientific journal, also available online. Its website provides both general and specific information about GERD and other gastrointestinal diseases.
www.gastro.org

### FOUNDATION FOR DIGESTIVE HEALTH AND NUTRITION

The Foundation for Digestive health and Nutrition is the foundation of the American Gastroenterological Association, separately incorporated from the AGA. Its mission is to conduct public education initiatives related to digestive diseases and raise funds for research in this area. It also provides grants to clinicians and researchers. The Foundation publishes *Digestive Health & Nutrition* magazine.

Info@fdhn.org.

### INTERNATIONAL FOUNDATION FOR FUNCTIONAL GASTROINTESTINAL DISORDERS

The International Foundation for Functional Gastrointestinal Disorders was founded in 1991. It addresses the issues surrounding life with gastrointestinal functional and motility disorders and seeks to increase the awareness of these disorders among the general public, researchers and the clinical care community. Its website provides general information about diseases of the gastrointestinal tract.

www.iffgd.org.

### NATIONAL INSTITUTE OF DIABETES AND DIGESTIVE AND KIDNEY DISEASES

The National Institute of Diabetes and Digestive and Kidney Diseases conducts and supports research on the diseases of internal medicine and related subspecialty fields. Its website provides information about these diseases.

2 Information Way
Bethesda, MD  20892-3570
(301) 654-3810
www.niddk.nih.gov

### NATIONAL HEARTBURN ALLIANCE

The National Heartburn Alliance was created to be a recognized authority that provides a community of support for heartburn sufferers by providing education about the causes and effects of heartburn, as well as solutions that offer them relief and improved quality of life. The Alliance website provides information about GERD, free brochures and information about support groups.

www.heartburnalliance.org

## NATIONAL INSTITUTES OF HEALTH

The National Institutes of Health began as the one-room Laboratory of Hygiene in 1887 and is now one of the world's foremost medical research centers. It is an agency of the U.S. Department of Health and Human Services. Available through its website is information on GERD, as well as information on a wide variety of health related issues.

9000 Rockville Pike
Bethesda, MD  20892
www.hih.gov

## U.S. DEPARTMENT OF AGRICULTURE

Among its other responsibilities, the United States Department of Agriculture conducts extensive studies on nutrition and periodically publishes the "Food Pyramid" that is frequently used as a guide to proper nutritional practices.

www.usda.gov.

## U.S. FOOD AND DRUG ADMINISTRATION

The U.S. Food and Drug administration is the federal agency that promotes and protects public health by monitoring pharmaceutical and other products that are available to the public in the United States. Available on its website is information about medications commonly prescribed for GERD and other gastrointestinal diseases.

www.fda.gov.

## Selected Bibliography

### CHAPTER ONE: WHAT IS HEARTBURN?

Carlson, Karen J. MD, Stephanie A. Eisenstat, MD, Terra Ziporyn Ph.D., *The Harvard Guide to Women's Health*, Harvard University Press, Cambridge, MA 1996.

HealthWorld Online, *Heartburn*, www.healthy.net/asp/templates/Article.asp?Id=1733, February 6, 2002.

Hogah, W.J., *Gastroesophageal Reflux Disease: an Update on Management,* Journal of Clinical Gastroenterology, 12 Suppl 2:S21-8, 1990.

Moraes-Filho, Joaquim Prodo P., M.D. F.A.C.G., F.A.C.P, et al, *Brazilian Consensus on Gastroesophageal Reflux Disease: Proposals for Assessment, Classification and Management,* The American Journal of Gastroenterology, Vol. 97, No 2, 2002, pp. 241-248.

National Digestive Diseases Information Clearinghouse, Gastroesophageal Reflux Disease, www.niddk.nih.gov/health/digest/pubs/heartbrn/heartbrn.htm., November 5, 2001.

**CHAPTER TWO: UNDERSTANDING DIGESTION**

King, John E., M.D. *Mayo Clinic on Digestive Health*, Mayo Clinic, Rochester, MN, 2000.

**CHAPTER THREE: SYMPTOMS OF GERD**

Lindsey, Heather, *Gerd's Treacherous Ways*, Gastroenterology & Endoscopy News, March 2002, pp. 32-35.

National Library of Medicine, T. Kamolz, et al., *Psychological Intervention Influences the Outcome of Laparoscopic Antireflux Surgery in Patients with Stress-related Symptoms of Gastroesophageal Reflux Disease,* www.ncbi,nlm.nih.gov/entrez/query.fcgi?cmd=Retieve&db=Pub Med&list_uids=94, August 27, 2002.

National Library of Medicine R. Fass, L Higa, A Kodnerand EA Mayer, *Stimulus and Site Specific Induction of Hiccups in the Oesophagus of Normal Subjects,* www.ncbi,nlm.nih.gov/entrez/query.fcgi?cmd=Retieve&db=Pub Med&list_uids=94, August 27, 2002.

CHAPTER FIVE: DIAGNOSING GERD

Jones, Michael P., M.D., F.A.C.P., *Diagnosis and Management of Gastroesophageal Reflux Disease*, Hospital Physician, February, 1998, pp. 15-27.

*Practical Guidelines for the Diagnosis and Management of GERD*, Primary Care Physicians GI Initiative, Volume 31, Number 1, March, 1999

Scott, Mark, M.D., Qimee R. Gelhot, PharmD., *Gastroesophageal Reflux Disease: Diagnosis and Management*, American Family Physician, March 1, 1999.

CHAPTER SIX: CAUSES OF GERD

Home Consult.Com, *Gastoresophaageal Reflux Disease*, www.home.mdconsult.com/das/newsbody/1/ctt93429575/26543/1.html.March 24, 2002

CHAPTER SEVEN: THE ISSUE OF DIET

Borushek, Allan, *Doctor's Pocket Calorie Fat & Carbohydrate Counter*, Family Health Publications, Costa Mesa, CA, 2002
Marshall Brain's How Stuff Works, Calories, www.howstuff-works.com/calorie2.htm., April 1, 2002.

U.S. Department of Agriculture, *Food Pyramid*, www.nal.usda.gov:8001/py/pmap.htm., September 9, 2002.

CHAPTER EIGHT: HEALTHY EATING & GERD

Altruis Biomedical Network, *RDA Chart*, www.daily-vitamins.com/rda.html., March 31, 2002.

Altruis Biomedical Network, *Vitamins and Minerals*, www.daily-vitamins.com, March 31, 2002.

Health World Online, Haas, Elson M, M.D., *Digestive Enzymes*, www.healthy.net/asp/templates/article.asp?id=1864, February 6, 2002.

Health World Online, Haas, Elson M., MD, Nutritional Program for Fasting, www.healthy.net/asp/templates/article.asp?PageType=article&ID=1 996., February 6, 2002.

Janowitz, Henry D., M.D., *Good Food for Bad Stomachs*, Oxford University Press, New York, NY, 1997.

Marshall Brain's How Stuff Works, *How Calories Work*, www.howstuffworks.com/calorie2.htm., September 12, 2002.

Reference Guide for Vitamins, www.realtime.net/anr/vitamins.html, March 31, 2002.

Rombauer, Irma S, Marion Rombauer Becker and Ethan Becker, *The Joy of Cooking*, Scribner, New York, NY, 1997.
Sugar Busters, www.aatkins-lose-weight-fast-diet.com/sugar-busters.htm., February 7, 2002.

U.S. Food and Drug Administration, *History of the FDA*, www.fda.gov/oc/history/historyoffda/default.htm., September 18, 2002.

CHAPTER NINE: EXERCISE

About.com, *Cardiovascular Exercise*, www.exercise.about.com/library/blcardio.htm., April 1, 2002.
Brody, Jane E., *Panel Urges Hour of Exercise a Day; Sets Diet Guidelines*, The New York Times, Friday September 6, 2002, pA1.

Levey, John M., *Gastrointestinal Conditions in the Endurance Athlete*, Practical Gastroenterology, December 2001, pp. 13-24

## Chapter Ten: Medication for GERD

AboutGerd.org, Treatment, www.aboutgerd.org/treatment.html, August 22, 2002.

Altruis Biomedical Network, *Antacids*, www.e-antacid.com, January 3, 2003/

Delaware News Journal, *Three Firms Join to Make Generic Prilosec*, www.delawareonline.com/newsjournal/business/2002/11/02threefirmsjoint.html, January 6, 2003.

Dermnet.com, *Antihistamines*, www.dermnetnz.org/dna.antihistamines/antihist.html, August 22, 2002.

Destination R$_X$, Price Comparisons, www.denstinationrx.com/drugstore/compare/asp?SubSub-CatID=154&BrandName=&Sort, January 4, 2003.

Doxycycline.com, *History of Antibiotics*, www.doxycycline.com/anti_history.htm., September 18, 2002
Drug Digest, *Promotility Agents*, www.drugdigest.org/DD/Comparison/New Comparison/0,10621,61-14,00.html.

Drug Digest, www.drugdigest.org/DD/Comparison/New Comparison/0,10621,8-14.thml.

Drug Digest.com, *Histamine-2 Receptor Blockers*, www.drugdigest.ord/DD/Comparison/NewComparison/0,10621,36-21,00.html., August 22, 2002.

Drugstore.com/products, January 2, 2003.

Ecomall, *Antacids/Acid Blockers*, www.healthwell.com/healthnotes/Drug/Antacids.cfm., January 3, 2003.

Familymeds.com, January 3, 2003.

First Coast News, *Three Firms Unite on Generic Prilosec*, www.firstcoastnews.com/health/articles/2002-11-02/health_drug.asp, January 7, 2003.

Healthwell, *Aluminum Hydroxide*, www.healthwell.com/health-notes/Drug/Aluminum_Hydroxide.cfm, January 3, 2003.

Heartburnalliance.org, *Procedures for Patients With Chronic Reflux Disease May End Need for Daily Medication.*, November 6, 2001.

Information You Can Stomach, *What are the Medications Often Prescribed for GERD?* www.acg.gi.org/acg-dev/patientinfo/gerd/info8.html., August 22, 2002.
Janssen Pharmaceuticals, *Aciphex FAQ*, www.us.janssen.com/consumer/aciphex_faq.html., August 22, 2002.

Mayo Clinic, MayoClinic.com, *Antacids*, www.mayoclinic.com/findinformation/druginformation/drugin-voke.cfm?objectID=0005, January 3, 2003.

National Library of Medicine, Decktor, DL., et al., *Effects of Aluminum/Magnesium Hydroxide and Calcium Carbonate on Esophageal and Gastric pH in Subjects with Heartburn*, www.ncbi.nlm.hig.gov/entre/qurey.fcgi?cmd=Retrieve&db=PubMed&list-uids=11, September 15, 2002.

PDR Family Guide to Prescription Drugs, The, Three Rivers Press, New York, 2000.

Pfizer, Medicines & Products, www.pfizer.com, January 7, 2003
Pharmacentral.com, *Antihistamines*, www.pharmcentral.com/antihistamines.htm., August 22, 2002.
Pharmacy.org, January 7, 2003.

TagametHB.com, *Heartburn & Acid Indigestion*, www.tagamethb.com/faqs.asp, August 22, 2002.

Therapeutics Initiative, *Treatment of Gastroesophageal Reflux Disease*, www.ti.ubc.ca/pages/letter3.html., August 22, 2002.

Three Rivers Endoscopy, www.gihealth.com/html/education/drugs/h2blockers.html., August 22, 2002.

University of California, *Medical Therapy for GERD*, www.ucdmc.ucdavis.edu/health/a-z/85Gastroesophageal/doc85drugs.html., August 22, 2002.

USDA, *Protonix Consumer Information*, www.fda.gov/cder/consumerinfo/druginfo/protinix.htm, January 3, 2003.

Walgreens.com, January 3, 2003.

World Health Organization, *The History of Vaccination*, www.who.int/vaccines-access/vaccines/vaccinesindex.html., September 18, 2002.

www.hcbi.nlm.hig.gov/entrezquery.fcgi?cmd=Rerieve&db=PubMed&list_uids=11.

CHAPTER ELEVEN: UNDERSTANDING YOUR MEDICATION

The Health Mantra.com, *Understanding a Prescription*, www.heartcarefoundation.org/02/0206/0206674.htm. February 6, 2002.

The Health Mantra.com, *Drug Safety*, www.heartcarefoundation.org/02/0201/0201453.htm, February 5, 2002.

CHAPTER TWELVE: COMPLIMENTARY & ALTERNATIVE MEDICINES

Arnica.com, *Natural Medicines & Homeopathy*, www.arnica.com/tips/tip5.html., November 6, 2001.

BBC News, *Herbal "Heartburn" Treatment*,

www.news.bbc.co.uk/hi/english/health/newsid_14930000/149316
7.stm, November 6, 2001.
    Center for Drug Evaluation and Research,
www.fda.gov.cder/warn/cyber/2002/DRSANallnatherb.htm., September 18, 2002.

    Evans B. Phil, Mark, FNIMH, Natural Healing: Remedies &
Therapies, Hermes House, London, 2001.

    Health World Online, *Naturopathic Therapeutics*,
www.healthy.net/asp/templates/article.asp?PageTy;e=Article&ID=7
17, February 6, 2002.

    Health World Online, Reichenberg-Ullman N.D., M.S.W.
DHANP, *Ayurveda, Food and You*,
www.healthy.net/asp/templates/article.asp?PageType=Article&id=4
52., February 6, 2002.

    Health World Online, Runck, Bette, *What is Biofeedback?*
www.healthy.net/asp/templates/article.asp?PageType=Article&id=4
51., February 6, 2002.

    HealthWorldOnline, Lewith, Geroge T, M.R.C.G. P., M.R.C.P,
*The History of Acupuncture in the West,* www.healthy.net/asp/templates/article.asp?id=1820, February 6, 2002.

    Medical Advisor, The, The Complete Guide to Alternative &
Conventional Treatments, Time Life Books, New York, 1996
    Natrual Health Web, *Acupuncture*,
www.naturalhealthweb.com/articles/synesael15.thml, February 6, 2002.

    Pyke, Rob, M.D., Ph.D., Dr. Pyke's Natural Way to Complete
Stomach Relief, Prentice Hall, 2001.

    Rogers, Sherry A., M.D.,  No More Heartburn: Stop the Pain in
30 Days-Naturally, Kensington Books, New York, , 2000.

Rosenfeld, Isadore, M.D., Dr. Rosenfeld's Guide to Alternative Medicine, Random House, New York, 1996.

The Health Mantra.com, *Acupuncture Introduction*, www.heart-carefoundation.org/08/0865465.htm., February 6, 2002.

Ullman, M.P.H., *Homeopathic Medicines for Indigestion, Gas and Heartburn: Natural Remedies You Can Stomach*, www.homeopathic.com/ailments/new/indigestion.htm., November 6, 2001.

US Food and Drug Administration, *Spices, Spice Seeds and Herbs*, www.fda.gov/opacom/morechoices/smallbussines/blubook/spices.htm., September 18, 2002.

Walkinshaw, Catharine, *What is Reiki?* www.eatonville.com/walkinshaw/health5.html, February 6, 2002.

Williams, Thom, Ph.D., The Complete Illustrated Guide to Chinese Medicine, Element, Rockport, MA, 1996.

Whole Healthmd.com, *Supplements*, www.wholehealthmd.com/refshelf/subs...?0,1525,10040,00.htm. November 6, 2001.

## Chapter Thirteen: Surgical Options

Klaus, Alexander, M.D., Ronald A. Hinder, M.D., James Swain, M.D., *Surgical Treatment for Gastroesophageal Reflux Disease,* Practical Gastroenterology, November 2000, pp. 11-18.

Videoscopic Heartburn Center.com, *Videoscopic Procedure*, www.heartburncenter.com/videoscopicprocedure.html, November 6, 2001.

## Chapter Fourteen: Lifestyle Changes

National Digestive Diseases information Clearinghouse, *Smoking and Your Digestive System,* www.niddk.hih.gov/health/digest/pubs/smoke/smoking.htm., June 23, 2002.

National Library of Medicine, McDonald-Haile, J., *Relaxation Training Reduces Symptom Reports and Acid Exposure in Patients with Gastroesophageal Reflux Disease,* www.ncbi.nlm.nih.gov/entrez/query.fcgi?cmd+Retrieve&bd=Pub Med&list_uids=80, August 27, 2002.

CHAPTER FIFTEEN: LONG-TERM EFFECTS

WebMd Health, Habib, Lisa, *"World Trade Center Cough" Identified,* www.webmd.com/content/article/1685.53424, September 21, 2002.

CHAPTER SIXTEEN: BARRETT'S ESOPHAGUS & CANCER

Barrettsinfo.com, *What are Some Investigational Therapies for Barrett's Esophagus?*
www.barrettsinfo.com.

Fred Hutchinson Cancer Research Center, *Barrett's Esophagus, The Seattle Barrett's Esophagus Program,* www.fhcrc.org/phs/barretts/plain.htm., November 20, 2002.

Gastroenterology Therapy Online, R. Srinivasan, R., et al., www.gastrotherapy.com/literature/commentary/c060101.asp., August 29, 2002.

Iqbal, Muhanned, M.D., et al., *High Grade Dysplasia/Esophageal Adenocarcinoma in Short Segment Barrett's Esophagus,* www.sma.org/smj/97aug11.htm., September 23, 2002.

Koop, H, *Gastroesophateal Reflux Disease and Barrett's Esophagus,* Endoscopy, 2002: 34:97–103.

Laiyemo, Adelyinka Ol, and Duane T. Smoot, *Gastric Cancer in the Minority Population,* Practical Gastroenterology, August 2002, Vol. XXVI No.8, pp. 13-19.

Mayo Clinic Jacksonville, *Esophageal Cancer,* www.mayo.edu.mcj/gastro/esophacancer.thml, August 29, 2002.

Post graduate Medicine Online, Gopal, Deepack V., M.D., F.R.C.P., *Another Look at Barrett's Esophagus,* www.postgradmed.com/issues/2001/09_01/gopal.htm., November 20, 2002.

Sharma, Prateek and Richard El Sampliner, *Experimental Approaches to Ablation of Barrett's Esopahgus,* Practical Gastroenterology, November, 2001, Vol. XXC No. 11, pp. 30-46.

Spechler, Stuart Jon, M.D., *Adenocarcinoma of the Gastroesophateal Junction,* Clinical Perspectives in Gastroenterology, March/April, 1999, pp. 92-99.

Virtual Hospital, Harris, Brenton L, B.A. and Kemp H. Kerstine, M.D., *Adenocarcinoma,* www.vh.org/Providers/Textbooks/EsophagealCarcinoma/06Adenocarcinoma.html., November 20, 2002.

WebGerd.com, *Adenocarcinoma of the Esophagus,* www.webgerd.com/Adeoncarcinoma.htm.

CHAPTER SEVENTEEN: SPECIAL CASES

Eamonn, M.M., M.D. FRCP, *Classification and Diagnosis of Esophageal Motility Disorders,* Issues and Insights, Issue No. 8, July, 1998, pp. 5-7.

Go, Mae F., M.D. and Nimish Vakil, M.D., *Helicobacter Pylori Infection, Clinical Perspectives in Gastroenterology,* May/June, 1999, pp 141-153.

National Library of Medicine, Oorenstein, SR, TM Shalaby and JF Cohn, *Reflux symptoms in 100 Normal Infants: Diagnostic Validity of the Infant Gastroesophageal Reflux Questionnaire,*

www.ncbi.nlm.nih.gov/entre/query.fcgi?cmd=Retrieve&db=Pub
Med&list-uids=89, August 27, 2002.

Olans, L.B., J.L. Wolf, *Gastroesophateal Reflux in Pregnancy*, Gastrointestinal Endoscopy Clinics of North America 4 (4):699-712,
October, 1994.

Rider, Dean L., J. Alfred Rider and Andrew K. Roorda, *PEG: A
Safe Procedure in the Elderly Including the "Oldest Old,"* Practical Gastroenterology, August 2002, Vol. XXVI No. 8, pp. 38-44.

CHAPTER EIGHTEEN: COSTS OF GERD

Beacon Healthcare Solutions, *ICD. 9. CM-Diagnostic and Surgical
Procedure Codes*, www.beaconllc.com/hcref/cclookup/icddescrip-
tion.htm., August 28, 2002.

Maryland Health Care Commission, *Diagnosis Related Groups*,
www.hospitalguide.mhcc.state.md.us?Definitions/define_drgs.htm.,
August 26, 2002.

Vann, Korky, "*Save big On Those Little Pills: Prescription Drug Prices
Often Vary Dramatically, So Shop Around, Experts Urge*, The Hartford
Courant, Tuesday, August 27, 2002.

CHAPTER NINETEEN: FUTURE TRENDS

Aymerich, Ruben and Steven A. Edmundowicz, Endoscopic
*Treatment of Gastroesophageal Reflux Disease*, Practical Gastroenterology, October 2001, Vol. XXV, No. 10, pp. 20-29.

BioTex, Inc., Research, www.biotexmedical.com/research.html.,
August 29, 2002.

Doctor's Guide, *DDW: Gatekeeper Reflux Repais System May be
Alternative To Surgery for Gastroesophageal Reflux Disease*,
www.pslgroup.com/dg/2157ce.htm., August 30, 2002.

MSNBC, *New Devices Promise Heartburn Cure*, www.msnbc.com/news/399068.asp?cpl=1., November 6, 2001

National Cancer Institute, *NCI-Sponsored Trials of Celecoxib for Cancer Prevention*, www.newscenter.cancer.gov/pressrelease/celecoxibupdate.html, August 30, 2002.

University of Kentucky, *UK Physician Announces New Investigational Acid Reflux Treatment*, www.uky.edu.PR/News/acidreflux.htm., August 29, 2002.

Virtual Drugstore.com, *Celecoxib*, www.virtualdrugstore.com/pain/celecoxib.html. August 30, 2002.

Winthrop University Hospital, *Photodynamic Therapy Sheds New Light on Cancer Treatment at Winthrop University Hospital*,. www.winthrop.org/pressreleases/pr200000626.cfm. August 29, 2002.

# INDEX

## A

Achalasia, 12, 38, 48–49
Acidic foods, consumption of, 42
Acupressure, 165–166
Acupuncture, 164–165
Acute gastritis in the stomach, 40
Acute GERD, 5
Adenocarcinoma, 49, 202
   causes, 209
   development of, 208–209
   diagnosis, 210
   symptoms, 209
   treatment, 210
Aerophagia, 98
Alcohol use, 12, 14, 15, 17, 40, 54,
   195, 205, 208
Alka-Seltzer Tablets, Antacid & Pain
   Relief Medicine, 140
Alka-Seltzer Tablets, Antacid & Pain
   Relief, Original, 141
Alka-Seltzer Tablets, Antacid and
   Heartburn Relief, 141
Alka-Seltzer Tablets, Antacid Relief,
   Gold, 142
Alkalosis, 113
Aloe vera gel, use of, 169
Alpha adrenergic antagonists, use of,
   43
AlternaGel Antacid Liquid, 122
Alternative and complementary medi-
   cine
   acupressure, 165–166
   acupuncture, 164–165
   aromatherapy, 169–170
   Ayruveda, 166–167

   biofeedback, 169
   Chinese medicine, 164
   digestive enzymes, 180–181
   distinction between FDA approved
     and non FDA approved
     medicine, 176–178
   food supplements, use of, 179–180
   growth and development of,
     159–164, 172–178
   herbal medicine, 171
   homeopathy, 167–168
   meditation, 170
   naturopathy, 168–169
   reflexology, 167
   Reiki, 166
   relaxation therapies, 170
   unregulated products, use of,
     178–179
   Yoga, 170
Aluminum hydroxide, 112, 122
Aluminum hydroxide, magnesium carbonate, 133
Aluminum hydroxide, magnesium
   hydroxide, simethicone, 134,
   135, 136
Aluminum hydroxide, magnesium
   trisilicate, 133
Amitone, 123
Amphojel, 122
Ampulla, 10
Amylase, 7
Anorexia, 31
Antacids. *See also* specific antacids
   active ingredients, 111–112
   application and use, 109–111
   dependency on, 21

# E

# S

Saliva, role of, 7, 18
Scar tissue, detection of, 33
Scarring of the esophagus, 201–202
Schatzki's rings, 17
Scleroderma, 12, 38, 44, 217, 218
Sedentary lifestyle, 41, 58–59
Serotonin, 43
Serving size, defining, 67–69
Sexual activities, relation to, 18
Sinus infections, chronic, 18
Sippy, Betram, 3
Sleeping on a flat bed, 41–42
Smooth muscle relaxants, use of, 43
Sodium bicarbonate, 112, 140, 141, 142, 143
Soft drinks, 54
Sore throat, 16
Sour mouth, 15
Spicy foods, eating, 14
Statistical evidence, 1
Stomach acid, production of, 10
Stomach, upset, 18
Stress, role of, 15, 40–41
Stretta System, 230
Strictures, 5, 17, 33, 44, 201–202
Sucralfate, 116–117, 144
Surgical options
  advantages of, 185
  Belsey Mark IV, 189–190
  cardiomyotomy, 190–191
  disadvantages of, 185–187
  Hill Repair, 189–190
  Laparoscopic Hiatal Hernia Repair, 190
  laparoscopic hiatal hernia repair, 186
  laparoscopic Nissen fundoplication, 185, 188–189
  Nissen fundoplication, 185, 186, 187–189
  recommendation guidelines,

182–184
  surgical myotomy, 190–191
  Toupet Partial Fundoplication, 189–190
Surpass Antacid Chewing Gum, 125
Swallowing, painful, 19, 21
Symptoms of GERD, 13–20. *See also* specific symptoms
Systemic diseases, 43–46

# T

Tagamet, 118, 146
Tagamet HB, 148
Tea, 53
Thermal ablation therapy, 234
Throat pain, 17–18
Timing consumption of food, 63
Titralac Extra Strength Antacid Tablets, 126
Titralac Instant Relief Antacid Tablets, 126
Titralac Plus, Antacid & Anti-Gas Relief Tablets, 127
Tobacco use, 15
Tooth decay, 197–198
Toupet Partial Fundoplication, 189–190
Tracheal stenosis, 208
Tums Antacid/Calcium Supplement, 127
Tums E-X Extra Strength Antacid/Calcium Supplement, 127

# U

UES. *See* Upper esophageal sphincter
Ulcerations, 5
Ulcerative esophagitis, 200–201
Ulcers, detection of, 33
Ultrasonic therapy, 234

# HEALTHY LIVING BOOKS

Healthy Living Books brings together recognized experts from the fields of health, medicine, fitness, and nutrition to provide millions of men and women with the reliable information they need to lead longer, healthier lives.

Our editors recognize that good health comes from healthy lifestyle choices: eating well, exercising regularly, and preventing illness through sound knowledge and intelligent action.

In this day and age, when fewer people are covered by health insurance and more face increased health risks due to sedentary lifestyles, improper nutrition, and the challenges of aging, there is a profound need for solid, tested guidance. That's where we fit in.

Our medical team consists of physicians and specialists from the country's leading medical centers and institutions. Our recipes are kitchen-tested for reliability and include nutritional analysis so that home cooks will find it easy to put delicious, healthful meals on the table. Our exercise programs are prepared by nationally certified personal trainers and rehabilitation experts. All titles are presented in clear, concise language that makes reading fun and useful.

## Visit our Web site at
## www.healthylivingbooks.com

Healthy Living Books has something for everyone.